The 4-Minute Miracle

Stop Dieting, Drop Deprivation, and Reclaim Your Sexy

Linda J. Curry

ISBN: 978-1-62747-243-2
eISBN: 978-1-62747-244-9

Disclaimer

The author, Linda J. Curry, is an herbalist and diet consultant. She is going to share knowledge and experience that may not be based on scientific proof, nor evaluated by the Food and Drug Administration. The information provided is not intended to diagnose, treat, cure, or prevent any disease. It is for educational purposes only, and is not intended as a substitute for the advice provided by your healthcare professional or physician.

What you do with this information is up to you. You may choose to consult a medical professional before making lifestyle changes. The author is not a medical doctor and the information provided should not replace the one-on-one relationship with your primary care physician.

Contents

Dedication

My dear mother, of course. Mom, you have inspired and engrained a focus of health from a very young age and I am forever grateful for where this path has taken me. Your guidance, support, and unconditional love is immeasurable. Thank you.

Introduction

Since you picked up this book, I'm going to assume that you're open to me dictating four minutes of your life each day. I suppose four minutes sounds doable no matter what it is, right? Well, now that I've got you thinking, maybe not. Let me assure you, these four minutes are not like the latest seven-minute workout that puts your body through extreme intensity for the longest seven minutes of your life. Don't get me wrong, I'm an advocate. It's quite brilliant, really. But I also intimately know its pain.

The four minutes per day I am encouraging happens to be the secret weapon for getting your sexy back and it came to me by accident. I realized the gold mine I uncovered when I was no longer indulging in dark chocolate at 2 p.m. or shoving handfuls of nuts into my mouth. And the all-too-familiar speed-eating-through-dinner routine. Yup, I owned all of those behaviors and in an instant, they were gone—all by accident.

I don't want to mislead you by promising some kind of miracle. In fact, the four-minute ritual I am advocating takes up little real estate in this book. But do not underestimate its power. For the most part, this book includes loads of wisdom and tips for your ideal health and vitality (not to mention revealing your sexy). You could say it is a diet book, although it is so much more. You see, the super simple four-minute ritual, if you will implement it, is sure to take your vitality to a grander level than you could ever have imagined. And this is why the title of the book is deserving of the word "miracle." This practice is powerful beyond measure. But it is completely up to you whether you will see benefit from it.

Do not fear this gem if it appears quirky and way too simplistic to make a difference. Some will decide to not try it because of its simplicity. How can something so simple be effective? Even if you do not take this gem seriously at first, read on and grab all the other shiny nuggets, as this book will still give you loads of wisdom.

Let's be totally honest for a minute. You and I both already know how to eat healthy. Kale, broccoli, and cauliflower for dinner and we'd be set, right? The problem arises when we're stressed, bored, sad, angry—or even happy, and suddenly we can get to the bottom of a bag of chips without blinking. This is where we lose our way. This is where we fall off the wagon every time. Those emotions tend to take over without warning and all our hard work and determination nose dives in an instant.

So okay, you get that emotions may be sabotaging your success. But the mere thought of working on your emotional "stuff" is unthinkable. I get it. All that "stuff" appears daunting and untouchable. But I am here to tell you that "The 4-Minute Miracle" is just that—a miracle. You don't have to unravel all the turmoil that planted itself in you to reclaim your sexy.

What if I told you that four minutes of your day could melt that "stuff" like butter and you can walk down the street exuding confidence? The melting that takes place literally melts fat, too, if that is something you care to do. Often, we unknowingly hold onto excess weight as a protective barrier. The 4-Minute Miracle can release that barrier. But losing weight is not necessarily everyone's goal. That is why this book focuses on reclaiming health, vitality, and your sexy.

Sexy can mean something different for everyone. Perhaps sexy to you means exuding confidence, standing tall, or speaking your truth. For some, it may involve toning your body, building muscle, or the capability of climbing a mountain. And for some it may mean releasing excess weight to reclaim health. Or perhaps for you it means defining your womanly curves. Whatever your sexy looks like, are you game to implementing a super simple four-minute protocol that can bring it on?

It's also important to be clear on what health or vitality means for you. Do you simply want to look good and exude confidence? Or is optimal health important as well? Do you want to live a long time, or do you also care about the quality of life you have? Get clear on what health and vitality looks and feels like to you and in the meantime, I'm going to assume you want to live a good, long, quality life, feeling and looking great. If this is you, I can almost guarantee you will benefit greatly from this book.

We will build upon concepts and protocols for reclaiming this sexy or vitality that you may be looking for. We will discuss common-sense food principles that may have been lost along the way. Or perhaps you never tapped into them. Regardless, I want you to connect with them once again, as it is critical for optimal wellness. This common-sense approach is so simple and effective that you can trash the "Google everything" strategy to find the next superfood or cleanse in search for that magic pill. After you learn the protocols, it becomes second nature for lifelong success dealing with food.

We will also ensure you have the wisdom on choosing the right food for *your* body, as one-size does not fit all. We have different goals, different genes, different vulnerabilities, different emotional trauma, and different lifestyles. By sharing concepts and personal stories, I will help you put the puzzle pieces together for your journey.

In addition, this book will lay important groundwork to shift your mindset around food and eating. You may have a certain relationship with food that needs a little tweaking before reclaiming your sexy. For example, do you ever feel deprived when you pass up a cookie? Or perhaps you eat the cookie as guilt engulfs your whole being. Deprivation and guilt will no longer be in our food game, because of their detrimental effects. You heard me right: deprivation is dead. Instead, allowing is the new way. This is not to say our diet will now consist solely of potato chips and cookies. But we will allow ourselves reasonable treats and even comfort food when we need it most. Turns out, The 4-Minute Miracle will cut way down on how often you turn to food for comfort anyway.

And guess what? With this protocol, you don't need your stinking willpower. Our emotions always kicked its butt anyway, so let's get to a place where willpower rarely comes into play.

Any chance you've ever tried a fad diet? Perhaps you've been dieting most of your adult life. Temporary dieting is finally obsolete in our new relationship with food. Through simple lasting changes, your new lifestyle is where you win. You already know there is no silver bullet to optimal health or your perfect body. It's time to finally commit to slowly tweaking your daily rituals for long-term success.

Did you know that healthy food can be scrumptious and satiating to even the cheeseburger lover out there? I will show you a super simple method to making healthy meals that are truly delicious without the need for recipes and without feeling deprived. You will simply love real food that is nourishing to the body.

And The 4-Minute Miracle will seal the deal. We will implement this simple daily ritual that is going to smash the stress-induced food comas, binge eating, and unconscious snacking that are all too common today. This is where the shiny gem resides. This is where it all comes together, and we transform your sexy once and for all.

If you have a serious reason for getting your sexy back, dive in and be transformed. If you think you are ready for The 4-Minute Miracle, the practice that will finally kick yo-yo dieting and deprivation in the ass, then let's do this. You deserve to feel and look amazing, period.

First and Foremost

Considerations

Before diving into chapter 1, I would like to address who can benefit from this book and give some tidbits on me, the author. Hopefully, this will allow you to decide if this is the right journey for you.

If you are someone dedicated to your personal growth and committed to your health, then read on. If reclaiming your sexy grabs your attention, then definitely read on. Perhaps you have tried diet and lifestyle changes but haven't realized the results you wish. Does your busy lifestyle often get in the way of your health goals? Have you been struggling to drop excess weight and feel it may be out of your control? And finally, have you realized that diet trends and short-term fixes are *not* the answer for your vitality?

This book will not give you a silver bullet. Instead, this book will tackle health and vitality from various angles and pull it together for long-term success. It is not an overnight fix. Although you will read techniques you likely have not considered before, this journey is about implementing small, practical changes that become ingrained in you for the long haul.

If you like to pick up books to gather information, yet rarely implement that information into your life, then you might be a bit disappointed. I say that because the title of this book claims a pretty big promise. And that promise is delivered only if you are committed to doing some things differently. On top of that, you need an open mind, because we will discuss protocols you may have never considered relevant in the past.

But I assure you that those very protocols just may catapult your health and vitality to record levels, not to mention revealing your inner sexy to the world (in only four minutes a day, mind you). If, and only if, you commit to trying something new and sacrificing four minutes of your precious day will you be able to experience these claims come to life. Is that something you are open to?

About Me

A little about me as an author and educator. I like to simplify things for my readers. In fact, this is kind of my thing, my *calling,* so-to-speak. I do the heavy lifting of researching all the geek-talk to bring you something simple, practical, and easy to implement. I will make suggestions in case you also enjoy geek-talk and want more detail on certain topics. I also put myself physically through the wringer at times in order to cut corners for my followers. It's not always intentional or expected but nonetheless, I have accepted this as my fate for the greater good. And I will share many of these personal health obstacles with you so that you can learn from my lessons and avoid similar trip-ups.

With a teaching background in the glorious world of food, I have been called "The Practical Chef." Although the focus of health takes the front seat, my cuisine is also *practical* for the busy person. That also means any recipes I give you may not be gourmet-restaurant quality. "Gourmet" is not in my repertoire by any stretch of the imagination. You will see things like delicious one-pot-meals, a quick blender soup, or overnight soaked muesli for taking on the road. I may also attempt to tweak your lifestyle a bit to prioritize precious time in the kitchen in a gentle and nurturing way. But I assure you, my suggestions are practical, always healthy, and quite tasty if I do say so myself. I take this approach with my students with individual health consultations, coaching, and customized cooking instruction.

I take a common-sense approach to eating and life in general. I tend to think big-picture and bring it to a practical level for students to make better day-to-day choices. Many solutions may not be your solutions, as we all have our own journey to walk. And although there are many similarities among us, there are just as many differences. My one-size-does-not-fit-all approach will leave room for you to experiment and make your own choices. I may eat an 80-90% plant-derived diet, but that doesn't mean you have to do so for success. We all have our own vulnerabilities, lifestyles, preferences, values and biases. This book will take that into consideration when offering suggestions.

In fact, this book is filled mostly with suggestions except where I feel we need to get real regarding lifestyle choices that are simply not health-promoting.

I will give you the nuts and bolts to common-sense eating and throw in a lot of other information for you to chew on. Some may resonate, some may not. Some may help to piece together your own health journey; others you may choose to toss. And I assure you, you will learn something new, look at things differently, and if you implement "The 4-Minute Miracle" for sealing the deal on your sexy, well, you may just transform your world.

Roadmap

I'd like to take a moment to explain the contents of the book in a simple way so that you know how to best use the gems to reclaiming your sexy in the most beautiful, efficient, and effective way possible.

Right off the bat, I am going to share some personal experiences as I introduce some common-sense principles around food and our bodies. These principles are essential to living a healthy, vibrant life.

Then we will dive right into our little miracle worker so that you can start this practice as soon as possible. It is recommended that you begin this daily 4-minute ritual as you continue to read. As your practice matures and develops, the remaining principles will become integrated for the best results.

After The 4-Minute Miracle introduction, we will implement strategies to shift your mindset around food and eating. This is essential as you begin to make shifts in your food choices and learn to love your kitchen again.

We will then dive further into common-sense eating protocols and principles that will ensure you have the wisdom to choose the right food for your body.

I will then share super simple methods to making healthy meals that are truly delicious without the need for recipes. But I will also share some of my recipe staples for quick delicious meals and snacks to get you started. And for those with busy frugal lifestyles, I'll share time and money-saving tips.

We will wrap up the book with emphasizing the importance of The 4-Minute Miracle to seal the deal. This is where it all comes together, and we transform your physique and vitality once and for all. Let's do this!

Part 1:
My Story

Chapter 1
Peanut Butter
and Sweet Pickles

Fond memories flood my mind as I recall mom putting out peanut butter and sweet pickles on a cracker. If you've never tried it, don't slam it. It's one of those things that just works for no good reason. This appetizer, using a crunchy Carr's water cracker, was served in the '70s and '80s in my home town of Sheboygan, Wisconsin. I learned as a child that peanut butter basically dresses up any meal from scrambled eggs to bologna sandwiches and happens to mingle nicely with a sweet pickle.

With no internet, my dear mother did her best to nourish her children based on guidelines from the dairy state, also known as the home of fried cheese curds, summer sausage, Johnsonville Brats, and Kingsbury beer. Believe it or not, most of my passion around food came from my mother and growing up in "Cheeseland." She worked hard to keep up on the health trends back in the '70s. You know, feeding your kids a big breakfast to make them smarter, preparing sauerkraut and pork chops for digestive health (or maybe just because that's what good Germans do), and eating liver and onions for God-knows-what. Or how about the good old-fashioned egg-in-a-hole trick, which basically is just a cute way to get your kids to eat eggs? Of course, at some point eggs were no longer good for us, but Mom didn't buy it and decided that moderation was key. At breakfast for example, she alternated between oatmeal, eggs, cereal, toast, and maybe a treat on the weekends—homemade donuts made out of dinner rolls (quite resourceful, that lady). Even though "Cheeseland" staples weren't the healthiest of diets, my mother had simple, good ol' common sense when it came to nourishing her family and I took notice.

I distinctly remember my mom making her own tomato soup and I can still taste it in my mind. It was bland, mushy, and nauseating (sorry Mom). I guess her tomato soup made her human in my mind. My sisters and I played with our soup until she left the room at which point we ran to the bathroom and dumped it in the toilet. On a similar note, my mother also gave homemade V-8 a try (which basically was her tomato soup chilled with maybe some carrots added). She remembers us girls taking it outside and spitting it out as we ran around the house. To this day, she says she has only one regret and that was making us eat Spam.

Mom did the best she could. Clearly her wisdom didn't come from living in a friendly town with a smoky tavern on every corner that sported jukeboxes, served 12-ounce beers in a glass, and dare I forget to mention, the ever-popular bowl of fried cheese curds. I know this lifestyle well, as my grandparents owned a tavern, The Tee-Pee, attached to their home. It was here that we kids danced to music on the jukebox and inhaled more second-hand smoke than any child should be allowed. Let's hope the benefits of the dancing and camaraderie compensated for any long-term lung damage.

To further emphasize the "Cheeseland" diet, rumor had it Wisconsin passed a law that apple pie must be served with a slice of cheddar cheese on it. Although I never actually verified that law, most believe this to be the case. Cheese was on everything. At any gathering or picnic (even today), one can find summer sausage, cheese, and crackers. Those staples alone could put half of us into cardiac arrest just looking at it. But it's so good!

I recall my mother drinking cola and not sharing with her children, as if it were a special adult-only, kid-forbidden treat. Perhaps my mother's common-sense knew that traces of cocaine (from the coca leaves) probably weren't good for her children's under-developed brains. Now that cola has high-fructose corn syrup or loads of sugar, this "liquid crack" is just as addictive and brain-altering, in my opinion. Thanks for sparing me, Mom.

My mother's influence taught me to always keep learning and doing better. With limited access to information, she did a great job tapping into her internal wisdom to nourish her family and bring joy to the dinner table.

Any *mistakes* made (are there really any mistakes in life?), turned out to be true blessings as I ventured on the path of healing my body and educating others in this crazy world of food. I cherish my mother's will and wisdom as well as the "Cheeseland" staples that have a special place in my heart.

Chapter 2
Signs of the Canary

As I step into my kitchen, I see, to my utter shock, a house guest dumping her smoothie down the drain. All the love I put into it, from harvesting the fruit, to pouring the pulpy goodness into fine glassware – all gone. My heart sank, as if a part of my soul went down that drain too. As I slowly step back into the bedroom, desperately hoping she did not see me witness the catastrophic event, it suddenly hit me as I collapsed onto the bed. The recollection of flushing my mother's homemade tomato soup down the toilet brought it full circle—God help me, I've turned into my mother.

Now mind you, at this time in my life, smoothies weren't even green yet. I was making fruit smoothies from the orange and pink grapefruit trees on my patio with maybe a banana thrown in. Trust me, they tasted good. I just don't think she appreciated the thick pulpy consistency. God knows how she might react to one of my green superfood smoothies today.

What I didn't realize at the time of the smoothie dump is that food being healthy does not trump taste for everyone. Even for those open to the smoothie revolution, most prefer to drink them, not chew them.

In addition, eating healthy isn't as common-sense as it may be for me, since I live and breathe food 24/7. Most people believe food manufacturers have their best interest in mind and food-in-a-box is for actual consumption. I've been there, believe me. It wasn't until I personally struggled to reclaim my health that I realized how critical food is—real food, that is. I have to remind myself that understanding the world of food is not always common-sense.

I am not a doctor and do not wish to interfere in anyone's medical care. I honor the medical community and what they do to save lives. But I also appreciate that they are not necessarily experts in preventing disease and living a pain-free, healthy life. I feel a strong pull to research, experiment, and educate to keep us on the side of health and prevention so that we can avoid the need for emergency medical care, because this medical care usually consists of medication and surgery, neither of which I'm eager to take on. Leaning toward fixing the culprits of our health challenges instead of "taking out" the symptoms may feel like a longer, harder path but the goal of lifelong vitality for the long-haul makes it worth the effort.

Along with the health research I am drawn to, my personal health struggles and celebrations (and those of my clientele) give me intimate knowledge and experience to share. I feel strongly about my purpose to be an educator of food and health. I have always been a big-picture visionary and putting the health puzzle together for myself allows me to assist others with *their* puzzles.

As an example of how my brain works, I observe the gross number of cholesterol medications people take today. Knowing that our brains *require* cholesterol makes me think we could be doing a huge disservice to brain health. The upward trend of dementia in our society alarms me; I wonder if it could be related. Another example would be the enormous amount of acid blockers in use. Most reflux is not an issue of too much acid but rather that it travels up the esophagus. These blockers may be helping to reduce acid reflux but they are also cutting acid production which is required to properly break down protein. Protein needs to be broken down into amino acids that the body can utilize. Without proper stomach acid, this is not done. Could this be preventing absorption of nutrients and wreaking havoc on the undigested food in the small and large intestines and associated with all the IBS (irritable bowel syndrome) today? I appreciate what the drugs are trying to accomplish, but many of them end up negatively impacting something else. I am baffled by the solutions presented to consumers today. These are some of the things a big-picture person thinks about in the shower. Connecting the dots of all the health trends and challenges facing us today is fascinating to me and is where I thrive.

Putting your own health puzzle together always seems a bit more challenging because we are in the thick of it. But I did manage to unravel mine (not without help) and will likely continue as things change. My personal health journey has lessons embedded I feel obligated to share. The food protocol changes I implemented over the years were life-altering. And my challenges became gifts as I shared my lessons with others and witnessed transformation. Improving your food protocol works—I am witness to that. With that said, don't feel that my food protocol is something I advocate for you. It is the underlying lessons that are important and implementing the right protocol for your individual situation.

You see, I happen to be like the "canary in the coal mine." If this phrase is unfamiliar to you, coal miners used to take a canary down into the mines and if there was any sign of struggle, or, God forbid the canary fell over dead from asphyxiation, the miners knew there was a health threat to them as well. It was basically a warning sign for the miners to clear out. I happen to be like a canary, which means I am super sensitive to environmental toxins, chemical fumes, electromagnetic stress, smoke inhalation, food additives—you name it. Some of us become the canary to show others the way. I have a love-hate relationship with this, as my journey will show.

I don't know what is best for *your* physical body at this time. But I do know that we have many commonalities when it comes to health challenges and can learn much from each other. Being a "canary," I feel an obligation to share my story, lessons, and gobs of research to give insight and hope to others. I also feel incredibly privileged to do so and appreciate anyone who shows up for this knowledge. Ingest the health suggestions, let it marinate, and see how it feels for you. The suggestions in this book are based on a common-sense mindset, listening to Mother Nature, as well as good old-fashioned experience—not necessarily advice a medical doctor might give you. Take the wisdom with a big chunky grain of salt and find what works for you.

Chapter 3
Immune System Speaks

How can some people live off soda and junk food? This has always dumbfounded me. It turns out the human body is quite resilient. Well, until it is not.

After coming to Arizona for college, I decided to stick around and enjoy not shoveling snow a bit longer. Many years later I found I was still hanging out and grew to love the lifestyle in Arizona. But I also developed some health issues that prevented me from fully enjoying the climate.

In my mid-thirties, I suffered from a chronic cough and wheezing deep in my lungs. This was probably the first time I saw my health degrade; I took notice. As I lay down to bed, the congestion would build and the cough and wheezing would persist, causing many sleepless nights. Anything that upsets my precious sleep is going to get my full attention.

After exhausting many efforts and buckets of cough syrup, a very potent anti-inflammatory "juice" came into my life just before my breaking point. I took an ounce two times daily of this powerful super-food and my body responded brilliantly, as I slept like a baby once again. I thought I found a silver bullet. But unless we can dig up the source of the pain or illness, no silver bullet will keep us healthy long-term.

After thinking I had fixed my respiratory ailment with this miracle drink, the next ailment appeared. The Arizona pollen started to take a toll. I would lock my doors and windows just to keep it under control, and even then, I would feel drained, as my body tried hard to fight the invaders seeping in. I often contemplated why some people are affected by the pollen and others are not. Why was my immune system so unhappy? Most give into their vulnerabilities as something they have to live with and support as best they can. I am not in the "most" category and refused to take medicine because of the long-term consequences of that slippery slope. And every time we mask a symptom, we are basically telling our body to shut up. Our body is incredibly intelligent, giving us signs of distress. Listening to it is a wise choice. Whenever I feel I can manage without medicine, I do so.

My health is priority number one – always has been. When I don't feel well, I am no good to anyone or myself. And so, I ventured out to my next move— herbal medicine. Some herbal remedies showed positive improvement in my health. Knowing the nutritional components of them, I kept making my herbal tonics and still do today—lots of stinging nettle for loads of nutrition and liver-detoxing herbs like dandelion root, licorice root, burdock root, and milk thistle seed to name a few. This is an important part of my regimen but didn't fully wipe out the culprit draining my immune system. I still hadn't found the source and although I was using natural remedies, I was still only treating symptoms.

Then, when I was going through an advanced herbal certification course, I met a nutritionist who suggested I take gluten out of my diet to relieve my pollen discomfort. Even though I didn't seem to have digestive issues, and couldn't quite understand the connection between pollen allergies and eating gluten, I was willing to try anything. My friend explained that 70-80% of our immune system lies in the digestive tract. And if gluten is creating havoc with my immune system, it becomes tapped out and cannot deal with pollen in the air. This explanation allowed me to understand that it's best to look at a broader perspective of the whole body.

So out went the gluten (mainly wheat products) for two weeks and guess what? My pollen allergies vanished – just like that! This is a common result for people when they eliminate a food sensitivity. I was beyond thrilled. Words cannot describe the thrill of finding and clearing the culprit affecting one's health. As a bonus, eliminating gluten also cleared my knee and joint pain, allowing me to finally hike again without knee support. On top of that, I suddenly had a six-year stretch without a single cold or flu (until I got a flu shot and it messed up my system and my perfect record). Taking gluten out of my food protocol really was a jackpot moment and to this day I avoid it. Any help I can give my immune system is worth the effort.

Turns out, wheat in general is not as healthy as most believe it to be. Today, wheat is grown, harvested, and stored in a manner that removes much of its health components. And due to the changes, wheat has much more gluten today making it harder to digest. On top of that, the plethora of pesticides used today degrade the quality of this once healthy food. And due to the abundance of wheat added to processed foods, people are consuming it often without realizing. Even if wheat is grown, harvested, and stored properly, it really needs to be fermented before consumption for digestibility. Today most bread is not fermented unless it is a true sour dough. We will discuss in more detail in book 2 of this series on gut health.

After the gluten realization and impact on my health, I was suddenly driven to learn as much as I could about food and its residual health effects. And that meant experimenting with more foods. Dairy was my next prey. Ridding my diet of dairy, including my cheese-and-cracker staple, was not an easy task. You can take the girl out of Wisconsin, but … (you get the idea).

Not only is dairy/milk in most processed foods, cheese is addictive, and I had fallen victim. Cheese is a solid substance of fatty, salty goodness that you can sink your teeth into. When you are hungry, a slab of this mystical creation can really satisfy. If you can relate, you know what I'm talking about. I do love a good challenge, however, and gave it a go. Buckle up, willpower—it's time to take you out of the closet.

Turns out, removing milk, cheese, and butter was a simple experiment that would end up allowing me to breathe through my nose again. A little history. Basically, when lying down to sleep, my nasal passages became blocked. I have a family history of sinus polyps, often removed with surgery. I knew I had them and feared going under the knife. Most people would accept this as hereditary but give me a bad gene and I'll find a way around it.

Turns out, when I took the inflammatory dairy out of my food protocol, the polyps healed on their own. I didn't even know that was possible. I could understand preventing them from forming but dissolving into nothingness seemed like a miracle. Our bodies do know what to do when given the right nourishment and eliminating inflammatory foods. At the time, I had no idea that dairy was the culprit. It was a fist-pumping moment, as most of my experiments were. Having full sinus capacity to breathe again was truly a gift and to this day I have never gone under the knife (or sunk my teeth into another slab of cheese).

Gluten and dairy elimination brought tremendous growth in my mission for optimal health. I was passionate to continue seeking and learning as I dove into more experimentation. At this point, most may think I'm going overboard with striving for health but understand this was my livelihood and how I give back to the world. My health struggles, experimentation, and endless research is nourishing in a strange but purposeful way.

Next, I went through a more intense food-elimination protocol to see what else might be creating turmoil inside. A food-elimination protocol is where you eliminate potential food sensitivities for two weeks and then reintroduce them one-by-one. After you eliminate potential culprits and suddenly bring them back, your symptoms will be exaggerated should there be a sensitivity. Through this protocol I discovered yet another food that was dragging me down. It has to do with the beloved peanut butter that I slathered on everything from toast to ice cream.

After abstaining from peanuts and other high-allergen foods for two weeks, I reintroduced peanuts first. I took a good scoop of peanut butter in the morning and felt nothing out of the ordinary. I did that again at noon and by mid-afternoon, I found myself unable to get out of bed from extreme fatigue. This little love affair I had with the peanut had been stealing zest from my life unknowingly . . . sigh. I laid there lifeless in bed mourning this love affair that had suddenly ended. It certainly was a bitter-sweet moment as I forged ahead stronger than ever with a shrinking diet.

Are you starting to see a pattern with my health journey? I have vulnerabilities that relate to the respiratory system: chest congestion/wheezing, allergies, sinus polyps, fatigue. Keep in mind, your vulnerabilities may be completely different, as well as your food sensitivities. The underlying lesson is that your immune system will be compromised if you keep eating foods your body struggles with. If you have physical distress, your body is trying to send you a message. And do not think your distress must be only in the gut for it to be food-related. Health starts in the gut and what you eat impacts your health, period.

In addition to providing health consultations and lessons, I happen to manufacture medicinal salves for skin issues (warts, growths, sun-spots, burns, bruises, etc.). Customers often ask if a salve will work on eczema or psoriasis, for example. I tell them yes it will relieve your discomfort but as long as you are eating something causing the outbreak, it will be a constant struggle. Unless you rid yourself of the cause, no salve will keep it away. Even my creosote salve that draws out warts and other abnormalities from deep under the skin, will not keep new ones from forming if you do not remove the cause. If you are serious about health and vitality, tackling your symptoms—even if you use natural remedies—will never get you there. You must get to the root cause and sometimes that means experimentation.

If you have symptoms of distress, ask yourself what you are constantly putting in your body. It could likely be a food you eat daily. It could be your environment in which you live or sleep (chemicals in mattress, carpet, paint, mold). It could also be a pet sleeping next to you. I find, however, that the biggest culprit that comes up time and time again is the food you are putting in your mouth. That has a huge effect on one's immune system. In fact, I was allergic to cats until I got gluten out of the picture. Your whole world can change if you simply stop feeding your body foods that cause distress and inflammation. If you remember one thing, remember that 70-80% of your immune system is in the gut; this makes it very likely that your ailments are due to something happening in there.

Please do not get discouraged by what may seem to be my very limited diet. I represent the canary and you likely do not have as many sensitivities as I do. And, with the secret weapon, The 4-Minute Miracle, you will be able to relax more with your food choices, as I have over time. But to be completely transparent, I steer clear of gluten and most dairy products, as I feel they do more harm than good. But understanding what is attacking *your* body is ultra-important. Some simple experimentation may reveal your answers. And often I find people already know what it is and are in denial (like my love affair with the peanut). We will go into more detail about how to perform diet elimination to identify your culprits in the next book in this series on gut health.

In this next section, we are going to dive into The 4-Minute Miracle practice that takes our relationship with food to a whole new level. Beginning this practice right off the bat even before we talk food protocol is key to the simplest, most graceful path to attaining your sexy. Take a deep breath, take a moment to just be here now, and open your heart for this simple yet life-altering practice.

Part 2:
The 4-Minute Miracle

Chapter 4
Your Why

What are you willing to invest to reveal and embrace your sexy? I believe when you picked up this book, you had already decided that four minutes was well worth the effort for not just your "sexy" but for life-long health and vitality. I am dying to share The 4-Minute Miracle with you so that you can begin immediately and will do so over the next three chapters. With a four-minute daily commitment to you in motion, reading further in the book will shift your mindset around food and tweak your eating habits to solidify this vitality thing.

Do you feel vibrant and full of life? Do you like what you see when you look in the mirror? Do you show up in the world with all the confidence and ease you desire? Is there anything more you'd like?

I'm not sure what your definition of sexy and vitality is. That is for you to decide. But if you're anything like me, revealing my sexy means walking with my head held high and exuding self-confidence in everything I do. Worrying about what others think of me is a thing of the past. What I do and say is elegant, graceful, and authentic. And the self-care that goes into this mindset naturally brings my physical being into balance, radiating the sexy within outward.

You don't have to be a "10" to be seen as a "10." If you feel good about yourself, you are going to exude poise and radiance as you embark on your journey with all eyes following your every move. They want what you have. And hopefully, you will be dying to tell them that your beauty routine is a mere four minutes a day of me-time.

Does this sound too good to be true? It should, because miracles are head-turning phenomena that just don't make logical sense. But I'm here to tell you that it works. For some insane reason, it just does. And you get to decide how far you want to take it.

The 4-Minute Miracle actually takes up very little real estate in this book. But the profound effects make it the prime essence, in my opinion. Yes, the diet and lifestyle nuggets can catapult your health in immense ways, but it is this super simple four-minute daily practice that takes the cake.

I haven't always exuded confidence in my life. I am an introvert by nature, comfortable standing on the sidelines. I am a true homebody who prefers to lounge in sweats and a t-shirt. I'd rather listen and observe than talk and participate. But somehow, somewhere, I discovered four minutes that changed my life. These four minutes are ritual now and what they continue to do for me is beyond miraculous.

These four minutes didn't rid me of my comfortable introvert nature, but they allowed me to see it as a strength. They brought confidence and acceptance about who I am and what I have to offer. Discovering that I was no longer stress-eating after implementing this ritual was a surprise and icing on the cake. You, too, may discover gems well beyond the intent of this book.

Will it work for everyone? I'm not sure. Some won't have a clear picture of why they want what they want. If you think that money and a perfect body will give you happiness, for example, you will be disappointed every time. Unless you truly think deeply about what it is money or that perfect body can provide, manifesting it into your life may not satisfy your deeper desires. What is it you really want that you thought these things might help with? And then ask yourself, why? Why do you want that?

What I'm trying to get at here is that when you dig deeper to become clear about what you really want and why, it's easier to stick to lifestyle changes and commitments. You have a carrot dangling in front of you reminding you why you are doing this. As soon as you forget your why, there is no point to continue making the effort.

Let's investigate potential whys. Do you want to feel sexy and confident in your body? Or perhaps you want to be healthy and live your days pain- and disease-free. But why? Why do you want these things? Is it to enjoy the people close to you? Perhaps you have children whom you adore and want to be free of health burdens so that you can be completely present and active with them. It is much easier to feel joy and fulfillment in one's life when you are feeling vibrant, confident, and sexy. Remembering your why is the carrot.

So, what do *you* want? And why do you want it? Keep asking "why" until you cannot get any deeper with your answer. In fact, journal around this. Take out a piece of paper or jump on your computer and start jotting things down. Keep writing and keep going deeper. When you determine *what* you want, then ask why—and go deep. When you have your what and your why, you will know it. The pencil will stop and you will take a deep satisfying breath.

That is the juice that will keep you committed to a super simple four-minute routine that takes no longer than tying your shoes twice. Are you willing to commit to this? Because some people won't. Some people will look at the simplicity of it and disregard its power. Some will try it once and think it's too silly. Some will try it for a week, see benefits, and still toss it in the trash.

We do this because humans (maybe women in particular), have been conditioned to be productive in order to feel valued. Most of us move through our days without even taking a deep conscious breath. This conditioning tells us that this productivity will ultimately bring us happiness. I'm here to say otherwise. Instead of rushing through your day, consider taking a moment or two after you finish a task to center yourself. Close your eyes for a moment and take a deep breath. The space between the moments is where creativity lives. It's also where your inner calm resides where you make better, healthier choices. This small space where creativity and possibility exist just may shift your awareness to more purposeful work instead of simply knocking things off the to-do list. And The 4-Minute Miracle happens to be one of these pauses.

It's likely that 80% of readers will not implement this practice for more than a week. I want to ask you a favor. Will you prove me wrong? If you fall in the 80%, you may lose out on the most life-changing, life-affirming benefits of this book's essence. Commit to this practice for no one other than you (and to prove me wrong).

With that said, I hold no judgments about whether you utilize the prime objective of this book. If I'm being honest, this is a book I, too, would gravitate toward. And I would see myself eagerly implementing new lifestyle and diet changes into my routine. And seeing benefit from them would affirm my commitment. But the other part, the fluffy feel-good part, is not as easy to implement. The problem is, it's not something I can sink my teeth into or physically hold. And so again, I ask you to prove me wrong and do something I wouldn't normally have done in your situation. Because I intimately understand and know its power, I am urging you to strongly consider this practice.

The 4-Minute Miracle is a commitment to you. A commitment to your "why." These four minutes is what will make or break your sexy. Will you join me and your fellow readers on a journey to get your sexy back—your mojo that is dying to come out and play? Let's dive right in.

Chapter 5
What to Expect

How often do you look at yourself in the mirror? I mean, really look at yourself? I'm not talking about putting on your make-up or styling your hair. I'm talking about pausing in the mirror and looking deep into your own eyes. Have you ever considered taking a seat in front of a mirror and hanging out for a while?

We are now diving into the miracle I've been promising. And yes, it involves you acknowledging yourself, in a mirror no less. Now before you slam the book shut, hang on and hear me out. Remember your why. I may be asking you to do something outside your comfort zone. You're certainly capable of this activity but the idea of it somehow sends people running for the hills. Let me explain further.

I came across this practice by accident. I have these things called mirrors in my home, and one time I decided to stop in front of one. My life began to change on that day when I realized I had been ignoring a huge part of me—pushing her down and continuing to be the productive "soldier" I had become. That productivity kept me from connecting with myself and continued to push my fears and limitations further within.

This practice entails a mere four minutes of focused compassion with the vulnerable part of you, or child-self, that has been hiding inside while you forge through the day. All you need for this simple act is a mirror, a chair, and four minutes of your undivided attention. I personally prefer the mirror to be full-length, with room to pull a chair up to it. Hand mirrors may work for you just fine, and they can be purchased at a drug store for around five dollars.

Before I give you the specific instructions for The 4-Minute Miracle, let me share my personal practice with you. I have established this ritual through trial and error to discover what works best for me. Here goes. First, I like to set some time when I won't be disturbed. After completing my morning "chores," which helps me to clear some low-hanging fruit to calm my "Type A" personality, I make a cup of herbal tea and head to my office. I close the door behind me, a signal for "me-time;" i.e., do not disturb. I choose my office because it happens to be a comfortable, relaxing, private place. I often put on calming meditation music to establish the ambiance. Feel free to create whatever sacred space feels good to you.

After the meditation music is playing in the background, I sit directly in front of my mirror with my feet flat on the ground and take some deep breaths. I focus on relaxing with each exhalation. Then, I look softly into my own eyes. I suddenly become very present, as the rest of the world drifts away. I make a conscious choice to be right here, right now, as though nothing else matters.

I focus on the person sitting in front of me, which I believe makes this practice easier than meditation. The mind rarely ever wanders, maybe because it is mystified by this courageous act and curious about what is going to take place. If I do find my mind wandering, however, I simply chant the words, "here, now... here, now. . ." over and over, slowly and deliberately.

As I gently look into my eyes, I sense my Inner Child feeling supported that I took the time to sit with and acknowledge her for a few moments. When I first did this, emotions surfaced, and tears were common. Many times, those were tears of joy from a child who is being seen after many years of neglect. I didn't realize I had a child inside of me who was simply afraid. She used to fight and resist my every move. Yet when I stopped to acknowledge her, this resistance slowly released as a bond of trust was formed.

It is important to treat the Inner Child as a child. The beliefs and fears formed in childhood are real. As would any child sitting in front of me, she deserves my compassion. I warmly show up and acknowledge her presence each day.

During this 4-minute session, I tell her things I feel she needs to hear on this day. It can be something simple, like, "I'm here for you... I see you... I am right here, supporting you... Thank you for being you... I am honored to be with you."

It really is that simple. You don't even have to say a thing. Just being with the Child Within will form a bond with her. Your intention and presence is all that is required.

This practice is especially useful first thing in the morning to get your day started off right. As I mentioned, I like to do it after a few chores are completed so that I can feel more relaxed. Or if your mind tends to wander at night, you may want to connect with your Inner Child before bedtime. This practice quiets the mind and halts the ego from thinking about all the things we said that day that we wished we hadn't, or the things we should have done that we didn't. Putting your mind at ease before bed brings a restful, peaceful sleep, which, by the way, is also a critical component of your sexy.

You could also consider doing this practice to interrupt your stress-eating triggers. For example, if you typically have a mid-afternoon potato-chip habit, consider incorporating The 4-Minute Miracle well before this trigger point. Maybe this is your ideal self-commitment time. If so, make it a rule that you have to do your practice before you can enjoy an afternoon snack, for example. In fact, make it your reward for doing the practice. Your brain will start to really enjoy your practice because it associates it with this reward. When you get up from your practice, a bag of chips likely will turn into just a few chips or perhaps even a healthier option.

Do you get the point? Schedule this practice into your day during *your* critical times. Experiment for a couple weeks with the timing and setting, but make sure you commit to it daily.

You can commit to four minutes a day, right? Based on the transformation I've experienced since I started using The 4-Minute Miracle, I would even sacrifice four minutes of my precious sleep if I had to. Are you ready to make a commitment to you? It's really quite easy to do so.

Recall why you are doing this from the journaling work you did. If you haven't journaled your why, do so now. Also ensure you have a space for your practice with a mirror. And soft music (without words) can help the ambiance.

Are you committed to living your life to the fullest, right now? Make a commitment to yourself to do so and start immediately – not tomorrow, now. Your Inner Child will be pleased to see you.

Chapter 6
Practice Guidelines

It's in the deep respect for you that makes it so super simple to control eating catastrophes. So now that you have your why and a commitment to yourself and your Inner Child, let's get this party started.

Go to your sacred self-commitment space. Take a seat, get close and comfy in front of a mirror. Go ahead, brush your hair away from your face or apply some lip balm – whatever you need to sit in peace with yourself. Now, look in your eyes. Just look, sit, and feel. Observe any emotions that come up. Look at other parts of your face. You should be acquainted with your face, since everyone around you is. Then get back to your eyes. Give your eyes some compassion. That person inside you has been through a lot—a lot of confusion, mixed messages, feelings that weren't clear or easily explainable. Acknowledge that Child Within. Be there for her. I bet she is pleased you are there.

Are you ready to get to know yourself? There are no rules. Simply go to the mirror and observe, feel – and simply be with you. Spend some quality time with yourself, four minutes precisely. Set a timer on your phone to ensure you spend at least four minutes committed to you. Acknowledge your Inner Child and be with her. Bond. Form some trust. This is the most critical part of your new commitment. Simply sit and be with yourself. That's it. Forget about anything you may need to do on this day. Just be there, completely. Give this child four minutes of your undivided attention. Commit to being fully present. Place a hand on your heart if you feel the desire. Show yourself that you are the most important thing in the world at this very moment and you are willing to take the time to just be with you.

This is a simple yet transformational way of gaining trust with your Inner Child and acknowledging her. Have the intention to acknowledge that person inside. She has been feeling alone and scared as you have busily gone about your days. But right now, you are here for her only. Your complete focus and attention is on her. Feel free to note any changes you observe after implementing your new ritual. Journal as the urge arises. And thank you for showing up for you.

The 4-Minute Miracle Instructions
(for revealing your sexy):

Find a special place where you can easily sit in front of a mirror, feet flat on the floor (or lotus position). For the first few days you may want to just sit and look in your eyes. After you get comfortable just sitting with yourself, pick one or two statements below and slowly and deliberately say them into your eyes. See how it feels to you. If something else comes up, speak freely to her. What does your Inner Child need to hear on this day? What does she need to hear to know you are there for her? Sitting with her may be all she needs right now. Acknowledge her. Do feelings and emotions come up? Be with those feelings. Feel them fully and have compassion for them. Here are some compassionate words I might say to my Inner Child to acknowledge her:

- There is no place I would rather be than here with you right now.
- This is the most important thing I will do all day.
- You are safe.
- There are no expectations here. There is no one to please. We can just be.
- I can simply be me. I am enough.
- This place, right here, right now, feels heavenly.
- Thank you for taking the time to be here with me.
- I feel so blessed to be with you.
- Thank you for being you.

Part 3:
Shifting the Mindset

Chapter 7
From Deprivation to Allowing

Now that you have incorporated a vital daily practice for your deepest inner wellness, it is critical that you shift your thinking around food and eating for the best chance of reclaiming your sexy.

Too many of us today have deep feelings of deprivation as we pass up the frosted cupcake gently calling our name. What was once cheered and celebrated as an infant now torments us to the core. Your Inner Child may still yearn for the joy and happy emotions associated with sugary treats. Unfortunately, your adult self seems to be punishing this urge. This is very confusing to the Child Within. And even when we do indulge, the all-knowing guilt trip kicks in. We just can't seem to win.

I'm a strong person when it comes to denying the forbidden cupcake. But it always comes with a price. The stress of this deprivation comes to a head in the sneakiest of ways. Granted, I keep my pantry free from junk food—only nuts, seeds, legumes, olives—you know, healthy stuff. But when my stress hits, you might find me not eating five or six almonds, but 20 or 30. They land in my gut like rocks, halting my digestion for days. Feelings of guilt follow—self-sabotage at its finest.

Deprivation and guilt have never resulted in health and vitality. The only thing it does is sends us off the wagon onto the gravel below. Are you ready to stop that cycle?

What if I told you to eat whatever and whenever you wanted without guilt? You'd probably think I was crazy. But because I keenly know how harmful deprivation and feelings of guilt are to one's well-being, including weight loss, I am going to do just that. Trust me, long term, deprivation fails us every time.

What I'd like to do is give you permission to indulge when you feel the urge. Grab that bag of potato chips when you're stressed, if that is what you're called to do. And head to the vending machine when you're pulling your hair out at work. But I urge you to continue The 4-Minute Miracle practice and keep reading to add more tips and protocols to your arsenal.

The opposite of depriving is allowing. *Allowing* is nurturing. *Allowing* means you are listening and responding to your needs. *Allowing* is kind and compassionate. Ignoring or denying your urges, on the other hand, is not kind. I am asking you to be kind to yourself as you would be to any child.

It's time to nix the downfalls of deprivation by eliminating it. And at the same time, you will implement the other principles in this book that will eliminate the emotional-eating pitfalls in the first place. But until you do that, you may still find yourself grabbing the chips or the cookie when you feel unsettled. You are not broken or weak when this happens. Listen to your needs and respond lovingly. You just don't have the tools yet to avoid sabotaging yourself. That's okay for now. In fact, that cookie alone will not have the deep consequences that guilt or deprivation carries.

Food is an easy distraction, which is why it is used by so many today. Food gives your body something to chew on, something to digest instead of recognizing the deep embedded "stuff" that we don't care to uncover. That "stuff" makes us feel weak, and frankly, we don't have time for it.

Will you agree to allow nurturing into your life, even if food is your only tool right now? Continue to make good food choices when you can, but allow some deviation when you feel the urge. Can you agree that *allowing* sounds like a better strategy than deprivation? Can you allow some indulging without feeling guilty or shameful?

It's time to stop kicking yourself to the curb every time you respond to your needs. I'm not saying food is a healthy way to respond but it is at least a response, so it is a good first step. Next time you feel stressed and grab one of your kids' snack cakes, you are going to be okay, you are not broken. Leave the guilt behind and chew every morsel with intention and joy. Indulge in the comfort it brings you.

Responding to your needs lovingly without guilt is going to move you in the right direction. As you build tools to avoid self-sabotage, like The 4-Minute

Miracle, your emotions will soften and you will find yourself calm and relaxed throughout the day making *healthy* food choices. And during those times of unavoidable stress that we all come up against, you can still comfort your needs without devastating impact. Do we have a deal?

Chapter 8
Diets to Lifestyle

Would you be willing to focus on health and vitality instead of weight loss? When we lose something, most often we try to find what we lost. So perhaps when we lose weight, subconsciously we try to get it back. And nine times out of ten, we are successful at finding it. Let's agree to nix that possibility and focus on finding our sexy (or health and vitality) instead. I feel that when we focus on health, excess weight naturally falls away anyway.

I cringe every time I hear someone going on a diet they've done in the past because of the "success" they had with it. Now I ask you, if they regained the weight and they need to do it again, did it really work? I think people believe *this* time they can keep the weight off. *This* time will be different. Diets are not working, period. It's time to stop believing there is a quick fix and instead slowly tweak your daily rituals for lasting change.

Whether you are prioritizing sleep, moving more, eating more fat-crushing vegetables, or tossing the boxed food, let's focus on slow deliberate movement toward health-promoting habits. Lasting lifestyle changes means you are willing to shift for the long-haul—not for thirty days. Avoid making a shift in your life that you are not willing to keep for good. That is how you will know if you are dieting or making a lifestyle change.

I don't mean to fault all the trendy diets out there. Many do have some amount of success. One positive about these diets is that many eliminate processed foods, which brings about positive change. Eliminating processed foods naturally takes out most gluten, sugar, flour, artificial flavors, dyes, GMOs, and preservatives, just to name a few. Whether a diet happens to be meat-focused, plant-focused, low-carb, or high-fat, they generally focus on "whole" foods --meaning, minimally processed. Even though the diets may contradict one another, the whole foods aspect is what I feel brings success, at least in the short-term, for many of them. And learning to live without the boxed food is a huge plus if it's a lasting change.

Taking a common-sense approach to your food protocol can avoid the pitfalls of dieting. It doesn't have to be rocket science. A diet consisting of 80% fat, like the ketogenic diet, doesn't seem like common sense to me, not long-term anyway (i.e. lifestyle). But most people are hoping that someone found the silver bullet and they want in! And eating a lot of fat sounds intriguing and well, delicious. Permission to eat fat? Yes, please. As a side note, I am a proponent of many aspects of the ketogenic diet, namely eating whole foods, greatly reducing sugar and simple carbohydrates, and burning fat instead of carbs. These aspects make sense to me. Unfortunately, most diets get too rigid, which may sabotage long-term success.

Another popular diet, The Paleo Diet®, for example, may show amazing results for those who are health-savvy. But for many, it's too easy to put focus on animal protein and get sloppy and forget to load up on vegetables. The downfall of excess animal protein without vegetables is, unfortunately, clogged arteries, kidney failure, gallbladder and heart disease.

A near-opposite diet, vegan, or plant-based, consists 100% of plant foods—namely fruits, vegetables, legumes, nuts, seeds, and grains. It sounds super healthy. Unfortunately, french fries, potato chips, and candy can be in the vegan category as well.

Either of these diets could prove useful. However, they may become too rigid to stick to them. If you implement common-sense principles, on the other hand, like loading up on veggies, reducing sugar and simple carbohydrates, consuming small portions of animal protein (if any), eating healthy fats, and sticking to the whole-foods concept, you will have better success long-term.

I'm not here to promote or knock any diet. In fact, my personally following a plant-based diet for six-plus years wasn't exactly modeling flexible behavior. What I do want to express is that using common sense and moderation is a good rule of thumb no matter what food protocol you follow. If someone gives you permission to consume processed sausage and bacon for breakfast every morning, ask yourself if that passes your common-sense logic. Just because someone else may have lost 20 pounds on a diet doesn't mean it's not clogging arteries and putting strain on your internal organs.

Instead of dieting, create a new lifestyle tailored to you. When tweaking your food regimen, work toward creating lasting changes. It doesn't mean you won't continue to make shifts, but they are never meant to be short-term. If you implement a change, it is not for temporary gain. For example, if you go on a diet that requires making vanilla protein shakes for three meals a day, ask yourself if that is sustainable. Is that something you are willing to continue long-term, maybe even for the rest of your life? And even if you are, is that healthy? Probably not. So don't even go there.

Now, going on a shake diet for a month may drop excess weight. But the point is, once you start eating real food again, that weight will come back and may bring friends with it. Plus, we already decided to nix the focus on losing weight. If that is required for your body to be healthy, it will naturally occur if you support it. As a side note, hormones can often be the culprit to hanging onto excess weight. I cover more on this topic in book 3 of The 4-Minute Miracle series on healthy aging.

If you have children in your household, this concept is of the utmost importance. Children mimic their parents' habits. If you yo-yo diet and focus on the scale, your children will likely follow suit. If, on the other hand, you practice a good, healthy, moderate food protocol, your children will benefit greatly even if they don't seem to gravitate toward healthy foods just yet.

One trick to ensuring longevity in your lifestyle changes is to allow deviation or a cheat day each week. This gives you permission to falter a bit and not feel like you've failed. There may be a health benefit to this tactic as well. When you occasionally introduce "non-food" into your body, your immune system and organs kick into high gear to filter out toxins and manage your blood sugar for example. This is good practice and ensures they are ready to go should you need them in the future.

Diets are out the window. It is time for lifelong healthy living. And if you try to do everything I suggest in this book overnight, you will likely fail. But if you do what you can today, and then do a little more tomorrow, you have the best chance of lasting effects. Focus on healthy replacements to avoid frustration. Even if you don't notice health benefits immediately, (although I believe you will), you know deep inside what is right for you. Your body is worth every ounce of effort to gradually and mindfully move toward balance. You and your family are worth it. Tell this to yourself during The 4-Minute Miracle practice until you and the small child within both believe it.

Chapter 9
Willpower to Habits

Where are your vulnerabilities around eating? My husband and I used to have the dreaded night-time snack habit. After a full satiating dinner, I would "feel" hungry again in an hour. I wasn't technically hungry and knew it was not a good idea to eat before bed, but the urge was strong. And when I would go to bed with a full stomach, my body needed to work hard on digestion instead of healing and regenerating (sleep is essential for maintaining a proper body weight, in case you were wondering). But somehow, self-sabotage would drift in around 8 p.m.

I used to count on willpower to resist my strong emotional urges. But unfortunately, willpower does not work long-term. A better strategy is creating new habits and even rules to stick willpower in the closet where it belongs. That is really the only proper way to deal with willpower for long-term success.

To create a new habit, I might integrate some nurturing activities before my snack-urge time of 8 p.m. So, I created a habit of treating myself to a nice bubble bath, or perhaps picking up a book around 7 p.m. These things are naturally nurturing to the mind and the snack urge ceases to rise. Jot down a list of things that comfort you (other than food) and start to incorporate them into your day—especially before *your* trigger times. I could also reset dinner hour to be earlier, like 5 p.m., and allow for a light snack a couple hours later. That would give me plenty of time to digest before bed. Brainstorm some ideas that might work for your own eating triggers.

Perhaps for you, the vending machine screams your name around 2 p.m. every day at work. Salty chips or something sweet is calling out to you, creating a power struggle in your mind. In this example, a new habit could be scheduling a walk with a co-worker at 1 p.m. Or maybe you could treat yourself to some social media fun or picking up a romance novel for a 20-minute break. The workplace can be monotonous, and you can break that cycle with something other than food. It may also be a wise choice to have a healthy snack like nuts or dried fruit at your desk, as you may need some nourishment mid-afternoon. Whatever the case, find something that will work for your situation.

But these niceties do not always "cut the cake." Sometimes we have a rough day and just want to indulge. And in these cases, I suggest you practice "allowing" and go ahead and indulge. Just know that these urges will come up less and less as you continue your four minute daily ritual.

I want to introduce another strategy of having "food rules." I have strong willpower but even for me, it WILL break eventually. Until you see the benefits from The 4-Minute Miracle, your rules become necessary to avoid having to count on willpower. So, let's talk about "food rules."

Most people do well with rules. The purpose of having these rules is so your willpower does not have to enter the picture. Let's demonstrate with an example. Let's say you have a food rule that you don't consume potato chips. You created this rule because that happens to be a strong food trigger for you AND it happens to be something you feel good about giving up. Now, if your partner brings a bag of potato chips to the couch at 8 p.m., willpower never needs to participate. You see, willpower comes into play when you have a choice to make. In this example, the potato chips don't faze you because you decided long ago they were not food for your consumption. There is no choice in the moment whether or not to eat them. Stick to your food rule and after a while, the chips really won't tempt you.

Or perhaps you create a food rule around meal schedules. If eating after 7 p.m. is forbidden, then it doesn't matter what your spouse brings to the couch at 8 p.m. You simply don't eat past 7 p.m. and you don't need willpower as there is no choice to make.

For this to work, you should establish food rules that include one or two trigger items that you believe would be good to eliminate from your food protocol. That may initially sound unrealistic. And it sounds like it goes completely against our earlier permission of *allowing*, but keep in mind, you are in complete control over what goes on this very small list. It won't fix every food challenge that arises—only your biggest triggers.

Let me give you a real-life example. When I worked in the corporate environment, Krispy Kreme Doughnuts would be left at the administrator's desk for sharing on a way-too-regular basis. The smell of this ooey-gooey sugary treat would permeate the office and it was nearly impossible for willpower or any other power to resist. On top of that, donuts happened to be a childhood treat which brings deep emotion with the scent saturating the office area.

The only way I could resist the donuts was to make a rule, namely, "I do not eat donuts." For my body, donuts are not food, period. I was making a rule that essentially stated I will never eat a donut! In other words, when the smell starts to permeate the office, there was not a choice to make whether or not to resist them. It was already decided before the donuts showed up.

I understand this may sound like depriving myself. On the contrary. I made this choice because I knew that if I ate one donut, I would have a hard time resisting them tomorrow and the next day. And I didn't want to go down that path. I knew the effects too many donuts can have on someone's health. In my opinion, donuts are one of the worst foods (loaded with sugar, fat, AND deep fried). With my predicament, I felt it was in my best interest to toss them out of my life. It felt like the only option to allow myself health and vitality. I probably went 15 years without ever eating a donut and I did not feel deprived. Donuts never really came back into my life because I know the health consequences of this food, but I did eat one a couple years ago when some dear friends found gluten-free, vegan donuts and proudly brought one to me. In that moment, I decided that this food trigger was no longer an issue (corporate life was a thing of the past) and I ate that donut enjoying every morsel. And it turns out I haven't had a donut since.

This really works. You may have to trust me for now. Keep in mind that I didn't include every unhealthy food on my food rules list. It was just the very critical ones that always seemed to creep into my world when I was most vulnerable. It was entirely possible for me to head straight to the vending machines when the donuts arrived to indulge in potato chips, but for some reason I didn't.

When you create your food rules, make them reasonable and doable. Start small, with a couple of trouble areas and see how it goes. Even if the donut arrives and you head to the ice cream parlor, this is still progress. You may recognize that you need to keep some healthy snacks nearby during challenging times.

And don't forget about rules such as not eating past 7 p.m. Or perhaps set up a rule that you cannot have dessert unless you go for a walk after dinner. This strategy is super helpful because it trains your brain to enjoy walking, as it will get a reward. And that dessert often turns into healthier choices over time.

Another rule to consider is allowing "unhealthy" indulgences like french fries, only if you make them yourself. You see, it's way easier to pick up fast-food fries than it is to actually make them, so the frequency of eating them will greatly drop. And this strategy still allows these indulgences.

I love my mother's rule that she cannot shower until she goes to the gym. How many days can one go without showering? I'll ask her and get back with you.

Decide where *your* problem areas exist and go from there. Create a food-rules list specifically tailored to you. Write it down, print it out, and display it where you will see it until it is second nature. Consider sharing your rules with someone close to you. This will help with accountability. You don't need them to police you. Simply stating them to someone will hold you accountable in your mind.

One final consideration regarding willpower. It is difficult to make healthy food choices when you are "hangry" (where hunger moves into anger). One way to avoid making numerous faulty food decisions throughout the day is having a meal plan. This will assist in avoiding some of the pitfalls. If you already know what you will be eating for each meal and snack, there are no decisions to make and no willpower needed when you are basically starving, standing in front of your pantry or fridge.

Until you have a kick-ass relationship with yourself, i.e., The 4-Minute Miracle practice, consider making rules that you believe are realistic and doable (see samples below). Remember, willpower simply does not work long-term. It only creates feelings of deprivation (and that is the best-case scenario when willpower *actually* works). Deprivation causes more issues deep within that you will have to unravel later. Make your rules and see how it goes. What do you have to lose?

Triggers and New Habits (samples)

Challenge/Triggers	New Rules/Habits
Need to drink more water	New Rule: Drink 16oz upon waking each morning before breakfast
No time for breakfast	New Rule: Breakfast is not optional. Idea: Prep soaked oats or chia seed in Mason jar night before
Mid-afternoon vending machine snack	New Rule: I never eat from vending machines. Idea: bring healthy snack to work (nuts, seeds, yogurt, etc.)
Nighttime sweet tooth before bed	New Rule: no eating past 7 p.m. Idea: Eat dinner earlier and make time for earlier snack. Create some healthier options that are still satisfying.
Fast Food temptation on way home from work	New Rule: I no longer eat fast food after work. Idea: Have healthy snack at work around 4PM.
I need to eat more salads	New Rule: I have one green salad for lunch at least 5 days/week. OR I cannot have dessert if I haven't had a salad. Idea: On Sundays, prepare big bowl of fresh salad greens and pack for work night before.

Chapter 10
Mindful Eating

Before diving into food protocols, we are going to address one more practice—mindful eating. Then when you do implement new food protocols, you will do so with more health-promoting intention.

Practicing mindful eating can be challenging, especially if you have any subconscious beliefs around food that brings out the race car driver in you (like me). But every time you can become conscious of your behavior, you can take a breath and become mindful again. The more you practice, the better you become and your relationship with food will nurture you beyond those stinking beliefs.

I often wonder if people who pray or give energy to their food before a meal digest better. It makes sense. They take a moment before diving in to give thanks and appreciate that which is in front of them. Even if your family is not the praying type, take a long slow breath as you look at your food and give silent appreciation for it. This simple act can take your stressed mind to a place of gratitude and just may transform how your body deals with the food.

Are you open to a little experiment on being present and mindful with food? Bringing your body and senses into presence is a gift you can give yourself at any time. This illustration will over-exaggerate a simple act of being present, respectful, and grateful with your food. Give it a try to bring more mindfulness into your daily life.

I invite you to go to the kitchen and prepare a meal, snack, or drink. I will use a cup of tea as an example. Instead of going through your usual motions of this activity, this time I want you to honor the cup, the water, the herbs, and the entire process. You will be with the process fully – your whole being engaged with all of your senses. Initially, you will want to exaggerate this process. And as time goes on, your presence will become second nature.

Look in the cupboard and pick out the mug that speaks to your heart. It will pop into your awareness quickly. Take that mug into your hands—both hands—and give it a little hug by closing your eyes for a moment and taking a deep breath.

As you pour water into the tea kettle, watch the movement of it and how it dances into the kettle. Water is a miracle all on its own. You can really sense the miracle it is when you observe its movement and fluidity. Take the time needed to appreciate it.

As the water warms on the stove, pick out the tea that you feel drawn to. When you have picked out the perfect tea or herbs, bring it up to your nose. Take a big inhale as the aroma enters your being. Allow your body to integrate with the essence of this gift from the earth.

Then gently place the tea in your mug. If you care for honey or another sweetener, dip your spoon into the honey and observe the thick gooiness and sticky consistency. Allow the honey to slowly drip off the spoon and into the mug. As your mouth begins to salivate, put the spoon with the remaining honey into your mouth and close your eyes. Fully taste the essence of the gift from this nourishing food. The communion of multiple aspects of Mother Nature produced this miracle of sweetness. Envelop this essence into your being.

As you hear the water boil, pour the hot water over the tea leaves to hydrate and awaken the essences. Lift the cup to your nose to catch a glimpse of this miracle. Stir the honey into the mixture as the sweetness permeates the tonic. Allow your cup of grace to steep and marinate only as nature knows how, as you warm your hands cradling the mug. Feel your heart expand with this experience.

Do you see how present you can be with this process and how much joy and appreciation exists when you do? And you haven't even taken a sip yet! Our natural connection with the gifts from the earth is within you.

Go ahead and take a sip. Relish the moment as you feel the warm liquid touch your lips, the aroma enter your nose, and the concoction wake up your tongue. This warm liquid slides down your throat and your whole body becomes nourished by that sip from Mother Earth. Ah, the glory in a cup of tea.

You see, people don't gravitate toward tea by taste alone. It is the experience and nurturing that is the real blessing. Without you interacting with it, it was just dry green bits of a plant until you awakened it.

You can have that kind of relationship with all food, animals, and people, including the relationship with you. You may think there is not enough time to cherish all of your moments like this one. But let me ask you this. When you are not present, what is the point? Isn't *that* wasted time? When you are not present, your time is wasted as you flounder through life. It is a grand opportunity completely lost. Without going deeper into the practice of presence I will simply direct you to my book <u>Pebbles of Gold</u> should you want to learn more.

Hear me out on this. Give this a try, bringing your appreciation to all things. Be present with each person and situation you experience. Listen to your life – fully! You are worth it. Your kids, spouse, friends, and neighbors will benefit. And you will have the opportunity to experience pure grace with life.

Section Review

- Start your 4-Minute Miracle practice and watch your emotions around food settle down.
- Determine your "why" for wanting health and vitality. Go deep.
- Slash depriving and feelings of guilt after indulging. Enough already. You don't need to deprive yourself any longer and it was not serving you. *Allowing,* on the other hand, is compassionate and giving to your needs. And when you allow, you can fully enjoy it, bite by bite.
- Determine your challenge/trigger areas and create habits to soften any catastrophes, such as having nuts or seeds at work before hunger strikes.
- Continue your 4-minute ritual to bring acknowledgement to your Child Within. Allow her to feel safe with you.
- Stop dieting and create healthy habits instead based on your individual needs. Take it one step at a time and start to substitute healthier options.
- Create food rules that tailor your lifestyle and challenge areas to put willpower (constant food decisions) aside. For example, not eating past 7 p.m. or avoiding vending machines in the workplace. Create a very specific list that you can commit to, write down, keep close, and share with someone close to you.
- Nourish your Child Within as you prioritize your time with her, pausing for four minutes during the day.

Part 4:
Common-Sense Eating

Chapter 11
Longevity

There once was a man named Bernando LaPallo who lived in my town of Mesa, Arizona for many years until he passed at the ripe age of 114. To me, this man was a great role model for common-sense eating offering him a long healthy vibrant life.

Bernando grew up in New York and his father, who was an herbalist/doctor, taught him to stay away from processed and junk foods like the New York hot dog stands. His father ingrained common-sense food protocols that Bernando followed throughout his long vibrant life.

I met Bernando at a raw food potluck in Mesa and even though eating 100% raw all the time is not something I nor Bernando did, we both had an interest in healthy eating; raw plant food is a big part of that. Other than an annual lamb tradition and fish once or twice a week, Bernando counted on the plant world to nourish him. He started his day with a good hearty green smoothie that contained greens, berries, and superfoods, including raw garlic cloves (what a trooper huh?). I do recall him mentioning oatmeal as well which happens to come up quite a bit with centurions.

Anything that supports digestive health (regularity in this case) is sure to boost longevity (see book 2 in this series for more on gut health). He ate lots of salads at noontime and often had warm meals for dinner. That is what I remember from talking with Bernando over the years.

His food protocol makes good common sense. He wasn't a stickler with any diet label like vegetarian or vegan. Instead, he focused on healthy whole foods with focus on the plant world. A good-sized breakfast, including some amazing green nutrition to start the day, makes good sense. Lots of raw vegetables in smoothies and salads ensured consumption of living enzymes. And cooked vegetables release other nutrients for easy absorption as demonstrated by a warm cooked meal at dinnertime with whole grains or starchy vegetables. This also will calm your body and prepare you for a restful night's sleep. I feel Bernando had good innate wisdom, built upon a solid foundation from his father's wisdom.

Bernando also used olive oil to nourish his skin—with specific focus on his feet. He felt that soaking his feet nightly and massaging them with olive oil was nourishing to the whole body. I love Bernando's mentality that we nourish our body from nature. My motto that I use with my own skin-care line is, "If you can't eat it, don't put it on your skin."

Bernando was also fairly active as a centenarian. I will never forget his advice on exercise and movement: "If you want to walk two miles when you're 80, you best be walking two miles now." Bernando was known to walk two miles daily without fail and didn't miss his walk even on the day he left this earth.

Bernando lived a long, vibrant life void of disease and medications. In fact, he claims to have never had a cold or flu in all his 114 years. Some may doubt his memory with a claim like that, but I believe him. Perhaps this is what a processed food-free life is like. He took great care of his body using a simple, natural, common-sense approach to health. He looked to nature and primarily got his nourishment from plant foods— both raw and cooked, with occasional animal protein. Having some variability in his diet proved useful. And it makes sense, does it not? Simplicity at its finest. Bernando's food regimen followed a common-sense protocol and I am inspired and blessed to have known him. He wrote a couple books sharing this simple wisdom of healthy living if you care to learn more.

Chapter 12
Vegetables Rule

Teaching a common-sense approach to eating and health stems from my upbringing, as well as role models like Bernando. Taking a more simplistic approach will ensure you don't have to rely on keeping up on a bunch of studies, few of which have validity anyway. And then you can stop listening to me, too, because you will come up with your own wisdom that is right for *your* body. Using a common-sense approach to health and knowing your body is key to this vitality thing. The super simple food protocols we will discuss combined with The 4-Minute Miracle will build a solid health-promoting relationship with food.

Let's introduce the most important and simplistic common-sense eating protocol in my humble opinion. It has to do with the beloved veggie. Even though we generally think that moderation in all things is a good rule of thumb, I'm veggie-biased. I think you can just go gang-busters on non-starchy vegetables. It's nearly impossible to overdo it.

I also like the general rule of thumb that plant foods have a starring role on your dinner plate, regardless of whether you consume meat. Meat can be acidic to the body and vegetables will help alkalize the meal. Veggies also provide the fiber that is totally lacking in animal foods, namely meat, cheese, eggs, and fish. The fiber from vegetables will help push waste out of your system efficiently. Oh, and veggies have an enormous amount of vitamins and minerals that are essential for you to keep kicking (not to mention a bunch of cancer-fighting properties).

Just for clarification, this "super simple" common-sense protocol focuses on vegetables—not necessarily fruit. Although fruit is super nutritious and delicious, most is loaded with fructose. I ensure a couple servings of fruit in my routine as our bodies do require glucose. And fruit (especially berries) has great anti-oxidants that deserve mention. But I also know that too much fructose quickly turns to abdominal fat and likely a fatty liver brewing on the inside. In the fruit arena, I feel moderation is a necessity. Whoever thought it was a good idea to lump fruit and vegetables into the same category on the food recommendation pyramid did not think this through.

So my focus here is on the king of all kings in the world of food—the almighty veggie. Learn to love them. Love them raw, love them cooked, love them smashed, blended, chopped, and spiralized; love them drizzled with olive oil and sea salt, love them broiled, steamed, and grilled. Vegetables are the key to health and vitality and I'm here to tell you, when prepared right, they can definitely satisfy.

Jumping into a plant-based diet and sustaining that for six-plus years gave me enormous practice at making vegetables taste amazing. And it turns out it's super simple to do. One of my all-time favorite preparations is tossing them in olive oil and sea salt, throwing on a cookie sheet and baking until tender. Just be sure to combine veggies that have about the same cook-time. Root vegetables (carrots, sweet potatoes, turnips, radishes) take longer than above-ground veggies (broccoli, beans, cauliflower, peppers), for example. I invite you to try it tonight, to ensure half your plate is filled with colorful veggies. Refer to the chapter on Kitchen Staples for preparation details and additional recipes.

Common threads for longevity across the world stem from locally grown produce, along with other food staples for that culture. For example, Mediterranean culture may utilize a slew of homegrown vegetables along with fish, beans and lots of pure olive oil. Japanese diets may utilize fresh produce along with small amounts of healthy fish and meats (condiment-sized), and fermented beans like miso or tempeh. In Okinawa, Japan, where people are touted as living long healthy lives, diet consists of locally grown vegetables (with emphasis on sweet potatoes). In fact, most people there eat sweet potatoes almost daily. I tend to feel that crops that proliferate in a culture are good for the people living in that culture. Don't think that you need to have a sweet potato at every meal to live as long as the Okinawans. Often, we run into trouble simply by trying to mimic the diet from another culture. Your DNA likely corresponds to where your ancestry lived.

And because DNA will change over time, you may also want to ask yourself what grows well in your climate.

Did I mention I'm a fan of veggies? Let me get on a soap box for a moment. If you are used to eating a fast-food cheeseburger, fries and a soda, there is virtually nothing in that meal to nourish you. Your body will scream for more food as soon as it leaves the stomach. You gave it nothing to hold on to and your body is yearning for nourishment. In addition, the burger and cheese offer no fiber and will cause your digestion to be sluggish. The bread turns quickly to sugar, spiking glucose, and the french fries will start to clog your arteries almost immediately. Do I really need to even mention the soda? What you may not realize is that not only does it contain excess sugar that causes your body to form fat around your liver and abdomen, but the carbonation in the drink halts the digestive juices required to properly digest your meal (if you want to call that a meal). Okay, I'm off my soap box.

I don't want to get down on anyone's meal choices, as I've eaten plenty of meals like that in the past. Well, not really, but I'm trying to relate. But I do want to explain some simple concepts that hopefully will allow you to use common sense when making food choices moving forward. The most basic concept I've been harping on here is basically, eat lots of vegetables no matter how unhealthy the rest of your meal is. Veggies can literally help prevent diseases such as cancer and auto-immune conditions. Vegetables are essential to any diet and guess what? You can prepare them to taste amazing for the whole family. Fill at least half your plate with vegetables, with lots of color and variety from meal to meal to ensure you're covering an array of vitamins and minerals. That is a super simple way to not have to be a nutritionist to cover your bases.

There is another super fun technique for remembering what foods are good for. Many foods look like the organ they support. For example, when you crack the shell of a walnut, the meat inside looks like a brain. And guess what? Walnuts are great for brain health. When you cut through a carrot, and look at the center slice, it looks like an eye ball. Most people know carrots are good for the eyes (high in vitamin A). Eggplant, avocados and pears all look like the womb and yes, you guessed it; they support reproductive health. Figs are full of little seeds and hang in twos when they grow. Can you guess what these little cuties are good for (men, hello)? Tomatoes have four chambers and are red. The heart also has four chambers. Yup, tomatoes are good for the heart and blood. Kidney beans look like, well, kidneys. And can you guess what they are good for?

And the list goes on. Celery, bok choy, and rhubarb all resemble bones, and they help with bone strength. If you don't have enough sodium, your body will pull it from your bones, making them weaker. This is one reason why I don't shy away from sea salt. Bones happen to be 23% sodium and the above-mentioned foods contain exactly the same amount. Is that a coincidence? Perhaps it should tell us to trust nature for nourishment. Citrus fruit tends to look like female mammary glands. And they benefit the health of female breasts and movement of the lymph system. Pretty cool, right? Nature really does have our best interests in mind and made it super simple to show us the way. Even kids can get this stuff. Load up on veggies no matter what food protocol you gravitate toward.

Chapter 13
What Food Is and Isn't

Let's talk more common-sense eating. As a health "foodie," this is my game. I personally experienced how food greatly impacted my immune system. I have suffered, persevered, and live today to share with you how very important every morsel of food is to your body and vitality.

This is really going to be so much easier than you thought. Because we are not going to dive into understanding all of food's nutrition and what is required for survival. What we *are* going to talk about is much simpler. It's a more sustainable approach to moving forward without having to be a health expert.

We will take a child-mind approach when it comes to recognizing food that is good for the body. For example, if it comes out of the earth, eat it. If it's too hard to chew and digest, cook (or soften) it. If it comes out of a box, toss it (it is not likely food at all). If the color of your food looks like a box of neon markers, it likely has chemicals added which doesn't even belong in a landfill much less your body. Are you starting to see the picture?

I understand this is not something you didn't already know. But it seems most people feel that convenience is worth the health risk. Or you may just be in denial. If others are eating it, at least we're all on the same playing field, right? When I was single, working in corporate America, I came home from work exhausted, ate a bowl of cereal and went to bed. My cereal was more the whole-grain variety than the sugar cereal, but still, not a health-promoting dinner. Eating food out of a box was easy and comforting—I know it well. This is also the time I was struggling with allergies, a sluggish digestion, and fatigue. My body was screaming for real nourishment.

Keep in mind, you won't fall over dead immediately after eating boxed food. Health degrades little by little until one day you get a wake-up call and realize you may not be here to see your grandchildren. And if you are lucky enough to meet them, will they be visiting you bedside or will you be pitching them balls? Let's aim for the latter.

Do you look to others for advice because you don't trust your own wisdom? Have you trusted that food manufacturers have your best interests in mind? Corporate farms and food manufacturers (and most businesses, for that matter) exist to make a profit, which may put consumer health in the back seat. Food manufacturers focus on staying in business and trying to one-up their competitors on taste, convenience, appearance, cost-cutting, and marketing for the biggest profit. And guess who wins? The stockholders win. This is not a consumer health-focused strategy. You cannot rely on food manufacturers or the FDA to have your back. You must be in charge of that.

Let me assure you that the number of unhealthy Americans today should be proof enough that convenience food is slowly killing us. If we remain on this track, one in two men and one in three women will get cancer in their lifetime. And if that doesn't touch you, maybe heart disease, obesity, or diabetes is your thing. The advancement of medicine today happens to be keeping us alive, but unfortunately along with it comes discomfort, disability, and many times financial ruin. Stress eating is super easy in that state and the vicious cycle continues. It is no way to live or to be remembered. Let's aim for the life where you are running circles around the grandkids, okay?

Instead of relying on convenient boxed foods, focus on items that have one ingredient. For example, raisins, carrots, walnuts, lentils (you get the picture), have one ingredient, namely the actual food that came from a tree or out of the ground. As a side note, whole foods also include animal products like beef, chicken, fish, or eggs. In book 2 of this series on digestive health, I explain the ins and outs of consuming animal protein—who should, who shouldn't, should we at all, and if so, how to ensure we are consuming it in a health-promoting manner. For now, if you consume animal protein, for health reasons, please don't go overboard—and buy sustainably-raised meat and eggs. It's important.

The ingredients you read on many boxes, on the other hand, are not likely recognizable as food at all.

Unfortunately, they are highly processed ingredients as well as added fillers, preservatives, sweeteners, and colors for consistency, shelf-life, taste, and appearance. Common sense tells me this is not food. That's all I need to know to move on.

All items marketed to us for convenience require examination. Look at some of your common food-in-a-box items. Is there an ingredient list on that box that you recognize from plants and trees? Likely not, so get rid of at least 90% of them. If that rattles you, get rid of 50% now, 30% later and so on. I am not going to go into your kitchen and hold you accountable. You have to want to do this for you and your family. Recall your "why" for doing this, for wanting health and vitality. Is it worth it to you? Only you can answer that.

What will it take to eliminate most of the boxed foods in your life? Perhaps you need to find some healthy foods you enjoy just as much. Trust me when I say you will. They exist. I LOVE food—*real* food, that is. This will happen for you as well and it doesn't have to be time-consuming. It may seem overwhelming to rid your life of convenience items that have saved you time and allowed you to stay sane in your hectic life. I invite you to start small and remember your commitment to your health and being a good role model for your family. Are you ready to rid your home of most processed foods, especially those with ingredients your six-year-old cannot pronounce?

Okay, so to break this alarming goal down to bite-sized morsels, pick a couple common staples in your pantry and find replacements. The replacement may still be processed foods but perhaps better than the ones you could not identify as real food. Choose a healthier grocery store and discover new and exciting products. And when you can, focus on whole foods. You might decide that in order to replace the frozen waffle, you may incorporate oatmeal two times per week in the morning or perhaps a breakfast sandwich with avocado, tomato, and egg on top of a gluten-free piece of toast. Can you start to see how this might transpire? Take it easy, take a breath; you can do this. We will be discussing later how to save both time and money to support your new eating habits.

How do you feel about the ever-convenient fast-food craze? I was hoping we could fast forward through this dilemma but just in case you aren't on board yet, let's go there. Fast-food is an obvious convenience pitfall. It may seem easier when you are on your way home from work, starving, and knowing very well that you do not have the motivation or energy to create a healthy meal at home. You don't need me to lecture you on eating fast-food. You already know it is not the path to getting your sexy back. What can you change in your life to avoid the drive-thru pitfall? Review the sample triggers and solutions from the chapter on willpower. Do you need to have some nuts around 4 p.m. at work so you are not starving on the way home? Do you need to make a rule that fast food is no longer? What makes sense for your challenge areas? Find solutions to avoid the pitfalls. If you look closely, you will likely find only a couple areas that bring the biggest consequences. Some simple tweaks can transform your health.

Are you ready to prioritize a life of health and happiness? Making conscious healthy decisions is not going to break you. Later we will debunk the time and money myths of eating healthy. And trust me, making an effort will give you much better returns than fad dieting and cancer treatments. This ride will be fun and as you make healthier choices revealing your sexy, you will become one to watch, one who inspires.

I invite you to start appreciating whole food that comes out of the earth and off trees. It's time to use common sense, with nature as your guide. Do not worry, you don't have to change everything overnight and I suggest you don't. Let these concepts *begin* to sink in. Be easy on yourself. Start with replacing the Pop-Tart with yogurt and berries once a week. Or simply add an apple into your daily routine. And appreciate the whole food for the gift that it is.

As you learn more food protocols and begin to change your mindset around food in the following chapters, relax into them. Do not feel you need to make major sweeps of change just yet. The 4-Minute Miracle is going to help you with the food challenges you may currently live with. Little by little, we are going to build a solid foundation and then seal the deal with our little miracle maker. Simply try to integrate these concepts slowly, eat simply (whole foods from the earth), and mindfully. You can do this.

Chapter 14
Breakfast Confusion

Let's get into common-sense eating around some controversial topics like breakfast, coffee/caffeine, and alcohol. It's easy to find evidence of benefits and downfalls of each of these. These areas will not have one-size-fits-all solutions, and you may need to do a little experimentation for you. Let's start with breakfast.

The confusion used to stem around *what* to eat for breakfast and now people are questioning whether we should eat it at all. There is a doctor currently on a road show explaining that the previous studies done on children eating breakfast were mis-analyzed. It turns out they used low-income families and gave kids free breakfast at school. Well, of course they are going to do better in school if they get food at least once a day! Without going into details on that study, just note that studies you have heard may not have as much validity as you'd hope.

You may have recently heard trending information about "intermittent fasting." The idea is to avoid eating until later morning or even early afternoon as your first meal. The theory behind intermittent fasting is that your body requires a longer fast period today than the 7-8 hours one normally gets during sleep. By continuing the fast for several more hours upon waking, your body will have more recovery time from all the toxins and stress you are exposed to. When there is no food in your digestive tract, the rest of the body can continue to heal and rejuvenate. Some health advocates suggest waiting up to 18 hours before your first meal of the day. If you eat your last meal around 6 p.m. that would put your first meal at noon the next day.

Keep in mind, intermittent fasting isn't supposed to be a weight-loss strategy if that is your goal. The prime objective is for your body to further heal and regenerate as it does during sleep. As an added bonus, you might notice more energy in the morning during your fast. Most people think food gives us energy, but the opposite may be true. We generally wake up energized when our digestive tract has nothing to process. On the other hand, after a heavy meal, do you normally feel like running up a mountain or hitting the couch? When your digestive tract has heavy work to do, the rest of your body tends to shut down, for the most part. Lighter meals and snacks can prevent this.

It's the nutrition absorbed from food that will sustain your energy over time. The reason you may feel that food gives you energy is because when you consume carbohydrates, blood sugar spikes. But what goes up must come down and you will crash, turning to food to do it all over again. That is mostly artificial energy.

Back to the question of whether to eat breakfast. The opposing theory—eating a hearty breakfast upon waking—will give your body and brain nutrition and energy to sustain your morning. That sounds like a good deal. In fact, many health experts may tell you to have carbohydrates, protein, and fat included in your breakfast, as your body will convert it to energy most efficiently (as opposed to the blood-sugar spikes and falls mentioned above). And this approach (as opposed to fasting) may be good advice for someone who has blood-sugar issues or weak adrenals. If you tend to get irritable when hungry, you may be dealing with blood sugar or adrenal issues.

Both approaches make sense, don't they? So, what are we to believe and do? My advice is simpler than you might think—eat when you feel hungry.

Most people aren't famished as soon as they get out of bed. Listen to your body and go about your day until you feel ready for breakfast. And in many cases, you may decide to eat something lighter like fruit or a smoothie first thing as it is easier on the digestion. In this scenario, your digestion continues to rest somewhat to continue healing and cleansing the body.

Fruit is okay in the morning if you don't mind taking a snack break every hour as it won't sustain you for long. Fruit, in fact, doesn't require stomach acid to digest and prefers to move quickly to the small intestine where the nutrition is absorbed and utilized for energy. Eating fruit in the morning is close enough to "intermittent fasting" in my opinion, as it is super easy on the system. This is a fine strategy unless you have blood-sugar issues as the fruit alone may spike your glucose. And it's likely you will be hungry an hour later.

I personally get hungry within an hour upon waking. And I don't feel like a big protein feast so I listen to my body signals. If I have the luxury of staying around the house that morning, I may graze every hour or so. I may start with something light like a greens-and-berry smoothie and perhaps soaked oats with blueberries an hour later. If I am off and running out of the house, I may eat a bigger breakfast with protein and fat to sustain me (a piece of my coconut bread with almond butter and avocado, for example). And if I have no time to make breakfast, I always have my "chocolate breakfast cakes" on hand, made with almond flour, black beans, and pumpkin sweetened with dates. I may slather one with homemade sprouted almond butter to add some fat. They are a great dessert as a brownie but healthy enough for breakfast, (find recipe on my blog at www.truebalancewellness.com). Unlike fruit and simple carbs, eating protein and fat will keep you from snacking all day.

Again, there is no one-size-fits-all approach to breakfast—sorry. Listen to your body, taking into consideration your lifestyle, and eat when you feel hungry. Do your best and honor you first and foremost. If you care to allow more healing of ailments troubling you, try the intermittent fasting approach. You may find you thrive using this protocol. Others will find it does not suit their lifestyle or goals.

Chapter 15
Caffeine and Alcohol

What does our common sense say about caffeine and alcohol? Let's investigate. You may have heard conflicting studies done at different periods of time. But we are putting studies aside for now because we know most are biased and tainted. The truth is, there are benefits AND downfalls of both. From a common-sense perspective, good old moderation applies. And moderation looks different to different people.

We all know that too much caffeine can make our body and mind a bit *batty,* for lack of a better term. And too much alcohol could lead to addiction and even alcohol poisoning. That is common sense to most, likely because you've played around those limits yourself. Most people know their personal limits, whether they abide by them or not.

You may perk up when you hear another study done on the health benefits of coffee that will justify your carefree habit. But you already know your limit and another study is unnecessary. If you remove coffee from your life for a day and you get a splitting headache, consider that your coffee "habit" may have crossed over the line of healthy. Use your common sense, not the next headline to justify your habits.

Recently, there has been talk of a "coffee gene." If you have it, coffee is supposed to be beneficial for you. I suppose you can get tested if you choose, but it is not necessary. Most of you already know if you can tolerate it.

For me, I cannot have much caffeine. Would you believe that I get a caffeine kick from drinking *decaffeinated* green tea? Yes, I said *decaffeinated*. There is always a bit of caffeine hanging around in decaf, and for me, it's enough to jolt me from zombie to a squeaky-clean house in 30 minutes flat. It hasn't always been the case, but in my health journey, I have found myself more sensitive to caffeine, as well as alcohol. Should I drink caffeine too late in the day, I am sure to be staring at the ceiling in bed that night. I get a good kick from dark chocolate as well as it contains stimulants including caffeine.

Alcohol is even more potent to me. If I were to drink ½ glass of red wine with a meal, I would wake with a hangover suited for only pirates. Everyone is different. You know your limits and you know when you are going over them. There are health benefits and consequences of both and the trick is to find the sweet spot for you. For some people, based on their physical vulnerabilities and intolerances, it can be detrimental. I personally like living day to day without the interference of stimulants and depressants. I don't care to have a roller-coaster day with spikes and crashes. I know what to expect with my energy for the most part, and without the interference, can better recognize when foods are not serving me.

There are many studies indicating red wine and other alcohol may decrease your risk of certain diseases. I tend to wonder if the laughter and joy expressed with friends and family during alcohol consumption may be more advantageous to well-being - not necessarily the alcohol itself. Social connection happens to be an indicator of health and longevity. Just some of my big-picture theories.

One of my great aunts lived to a healthy age well past life expectancy. She was a stern, speak-your-truth kind of woman. She had one beer every day and claimed it did her body good. I believe her. One drink a day is not good medicinal advice for *my* body, but for some people, that alcohol may kill some harmful bacteria from food you are eating or viruses you may have picked up. It may also assist the digestive process with an animal-protein diet. There are many factors that may contribute to benefits and downfalls of alcohol.

Another consideration is that alcohol may not be held to the same standards as 20 years ago. Take beer, for example. In the past, quality beer was brewed and fermented with a variety of healthy grains. Today, our grain is grown, harvested, and stored differently. Manufacturers often use cheaper grain and less variety in making beer today. In these cases, this alcohol will actually harm the good bacteria in your gut. On a positive note, some craft beers are using wild-yeast ferments and still use good practices. If you are a beer drinker, consider the craft beers and ensure you replenish those good bugs daily with probiotics and cultured foods like yogurt, kefir, and sauerkraut.

Again, we don't have a one-size fits all approach to caffeine and alcohol. If you really sit down and think about it, you will find your sweet spot where you thrive best. And if it's time to reset your body, eliminating it for a week may do the trick.

Chapter 16
Honorable Mentions

I'd like to spotlight some common deficiencies today. These deficiencies are likely due to weak soil with commercial farming, consumption of processed foods, or simply a compromised digestive system. You may consider getting tested if you feel you are nutrient deficient.

The first honorable mention is vitamin D3. We get vitamin D2 from food, but except in the case of some fish, food doesn't naturally contain vitamin D3, unless it is fortified with it. D3 is absorbed naturally through our skin from sun exposure. There are a couple common sense reasons why we may not be absorbing D3 like we have in the past. One is sun block. Although I don't advise you getting sun burned, I'm simply stating that if you're blocking your skin from the sun, you may not get sufficient vitamin D3 unless you are supplementing. And it takes approximately 48 hours for the vitamin to absorb fully into your blood stream from your skin's surface. Harsh soaps used today may wash the vitamin from your skin before absorption occurs. Personally, I feel you don't need soap on all areas of your body every day. Unless you are quite dirty, warm water does just fine. Natural home-made soaps without harsh chemicals are another option. If supplementation is a consideration for you, I prefer a sub-lingual form of D3 that dissolves under the tongue. It doesn't have to go through a compromised digestive system to be assimilated. As a fat-soluble vitamin, ensure you are consuming fat when taking it.

Another sub-lingual supplement I take is Vitamin B12 due to the high plant-based food protocol I follow. B12 is found in animal products and in plant-foods if fortified. There are some plant-foods that technically have B12 but may not be as bioavailable to the body as with animal protein. Remember, it's not about the foods you eat but more about the nutrition you absorb. Even carnivores are often deficient in B12 due to compromised digestive systems. This is something I personally get tested for on a regular basis.

Magnesium is yet another common deficiency (some say upwards of 70-80% of Americans don't get enough). According to one of my favorite doctors, Dr. Axe, doctor of natural medicine and nutritionist (draxe.com), foods high in magnesium include: spinach, Swiss chard, pumpkin seeds (pepitas), yogurt/kefir, almonds, black beans, avocado, figs, dark chocolate and bananas. But it's hard to know if you are getting enough even by incorporating these foods.

Magnesium citrate powder to the rescue. It's great for repairing muscles, relaxing the body, and helping to loosen stools (should constipation be an issue). I love to mix it with some buffered vitamin C (has added minerals) with a drop of Stevia and warm water for a nice evening drink before bed. Soaking in an Epsom salt bath is another way to absorb magnesium. Be sure to avoid adding soap to the bath when using Epsom salts as it will counteract the effects. In addition, try to stay in the bath until it begins to cool off again for full absorption. You can also find magnesium oil to put on your body after a warm shower or bath. These are great ways to increase your magnesium, especially if you are not consuming and absorbing it from food.

There seem to be a lot of women with thyroid issues today. And although I will dive into this challenge more in book 3 of this series on healthy aging, it makes sense to mention sea vegetables. I'm talking about sea weed such as kelp, nori, wakame, and hijiki, among others. Our bodies absorb the iodine in sea vegetables much better than that found in table salt. With all the table salt used in processed and restaurant foods today, it is not a matter of whether one consumes enough iodine. It does have to do with the type and whether the body can utilize it. I will let your doctor talk to you about how to best take care of thyroid disease but wanted to mention an easy whole food to incorporate into one's diet. I love having dried wakame and nori on hand to throw in a bowl of soup.

Turmeric is all the rage today and also deserves mention. An element in turmeric, curcumin, is the most anti-inflammatory food substance known. If you have health issues, it is likely you have inflammation. And using a natural whole food is a great way to manage it. I love to make turmeric tea using 1/2 teaspoon of turmeric (dried or fresh), 1/4 teaspoon ginger, a dash of black pepper, 1 tablespoon lemon, 1 teaspoon of honey, and a dash of coconut oil in eight ounces of hot water. Vary the recipe for your taste but keep in mind the anti-inflammatory effects multiply when you add black pepper and a healthy fat to the root herb. In addition, I use red curry (has turmeric) in many of my dishes. I guess you are what you eat (my last name is Curry after all).

I must mention probiotics due to the importance of good bacteria on overall health (more and more research confirming this). Although it is not easy to ensure you are getting a good quality probiotic with live active bacteria that will actually reach the colon, it still makes sense to take one as insurance especially if you are not consuming fermented foods. Take on an empty stomach daily to improve your chances of the bacteria reaching the colon. More on this subject in book two of the series, which is dedicated to gut health.

A good quality multi-vitamin is also good insurance to fill in any gaps your diet lacks. And be sure to check the nutrients mentioned above as your multi-vitamin may already contain them (D3, B12, etc.).

It is important to identify and take care of any nutrient deficiencies. Everybody is different, and your vulnerabilities may warrant a different supplementation protocol. I encourage you to get a good blood panel done to see where your marks lie. I also encourage finding a naturopath or medical doctor practicing functional medicine to support and guide your efforts.

Section Review

- How active would you like to be when you are 80 years old? Are you doing those things today? If not, incorporate them before it's too late.
- Consider a new love affair with the all-mighty vegetable assuring plenty of color for an array of nutrition.
- Eat real food that comes from the earth. Boxed food just isn't fuel for the body and is likely zapping your vitality little by little.
- Acknowledge your food-challenge areas and incorporate new habits to avoid the pitfalls. For example, having some nuts at 4 p.m. at work to avoid temptation of fast food on the way home.
- Create a meal plan the night before to avoid willpower coming into play when you are hungry and stressed.
- Intermittent fasting is something to consider to allow the body to continue healing and rejuvenating after sleep.
- Continue your 4-Minute Miracle practice daily to soften your stress-eating emotions and to solidify your new healthy habits.

Part 5:
Your Kitchen

Chapter 17
Time Saving

If you're choosing to live with a common-sense approach to health, and ridding your life of most processed foods, you may feel that it is going to take a lot of time to prepare meals. But I beg to differ. After you get into a rhythm, you are going to see how easy and delicious your life becomes in the kitchen. Take it one step at a time.

Before diving into the time-saving tips, I want to set some expectations. Kind of a good news, bad news thing. The bad news is that yes, you will be spending more time in the kitchen, so you might as well get cozy in there. Zapping a Lean Pockets® in the microwave for one minute is going to be faster and cheaper than creating a gorgeous stew for four. I am not going to argue with you on that. You ARE going to be spending more time grocery shopping, preparing food, and cleaning dishes with this new lifestyle. The good news is that you will be rewarded generously with your health, mood, and vitality—not to mention your sexy.

And I have some even better news to go with it. There are things in our lives that actually feed energy reserves. Like taking a stroll in nature, getting on the floor to talk to your child about something important, or working on that creative idea that burns inside of you. The activity of cooking a meal may seem like it is taking from your reserves after a hard day's work, but that is about to change. When you become committed AND present in the kitchen, the time you spend caring for your health and that of your family is going to feed your energy reserves. Please trust me on this. It happens. I know you may be getting home today from work exhausted and the mere thought of cooking a meal feels impossible. But let me assure you this will change. And besides, you really don't have a choice in the matter if you are committed to your health.

In order for activities to feed energy reserves they must be done with honor and presence. If you approach it as an obligation and simply focus on finishing so you can get onto the next thing, you will struggle. But if you approach this with intention, become fully engaged, it will add to your reserves—I promise. Please try this next time you step into the kitchen.

What does stepping into your kitchen with presence and purpose look like? Well, it starts with pausing, taking a deep breath, and feeling your feet upon the floor. Pausing for just a moment will ground you as you shift your focus to the here and now. Creating a beautiful meal becomes easy and even enjoyable. Forget about the other things you need to get done while you are preparing this meal. Move slowly with intention and focus and watch your energy replenish. I will dive deeper into the topic of presence in a later chapter.

If you're not convinced yet about spending extra quality time with your apron and freshly sharpened knife, let me ask you this. The time saved on zapping a frozen meal in the microwave will be used for what activity exactly? Watching TV perhaps to de-stress from the day? Or maybe you would have more time to clean the house and do some needed laundry? Maybe you could even help your children with their homework. Those are all great things, believe me. But if these are your excuses, I invite you to look at each one and decide where your health (and that of your family's), lies in relation to each of them.

And guess what? It's entirely possible to get your spouse and/or kids to help fold laundry or agree to do dishes with your new commitment to the family's health and vitality. Would you believe it if I told you my husband does the dishes every night without fail? This is our agreement. And men seem to love having jobs. If I get very specific on what I'd like him to do for me and give him another job title, I no longer need to ask. He just does it like clockwork every night. When I expressed how nice it is to wake up each morning to a clean kitchen, it sealed the deal for him. He wants to contribute and appreciates the effort I put into our health. Maybe I just have a super amazing husband - yes, that is true. But I encourage you to try soliciting help.

If you picked up this book, I bet you have prioritized your health and are eager to dive in. In the next chapter, you will find recipe and cooking staples. For now, here are some simple tips to keep your time in the kitchen concise, enjoyable, affordable, and practical.

- Start your day by loading up the blender with nutrient-dense whole foods. Pour into a jar and take on the road as needed.
- Chop vegetables in advance. When making a meal, chop extra for tomorrow for a two-minute meal prep. Store extra in freezer to preserve for soups or stews.
- Cook more grains or legumes than you need and store leftovers for quick reheat for another meal.
- Buy organic frozen vegetables to have on hand when you're out of fresh.
- Consider a pressure cooker to reduce cooking time and preserve nutrients.
- Eating simple raw dishes can save lots of time and give you loads of nutrition. Consider blender soup, smoothies, a nut paté and/or protein balls. Lots of delicious recipes online including on my blog (www.TrueBalanceWellness.com)
- Pre-make cultured vegetables like sauerkraut—adds good bacteria, is nutrient-dense, alkalizes your meals, adds a good crunch and keeps for months in the fridge.
- Keep grocery list on fridge. When running low on a staple, write it down. Shopping becomes super easy.
- Plan one day per week to go to the Farmers Market and grocery store to keep things fresh and nutritious.

- Make a large bowl of salad greens to keep in fridge for days.
- When using your food processor or blender, decide what else you can make so you can rinse and use again before washing. For example, after making a smoothie for breakfast, make a chilled veggie soup for lunch and store in Mason jar. Find recipes in chapter on Kitchen Staples and Recipes.
- Have the right tools in your kitchen. A mandolin for easy slicing, food processor for bigger jobs, blender, hand immersion blender (for salad dressings, pureeing soups, etc.).
- Make marinara or pesto ahead of time and freeze small batches.
- To avoid peeling garlic for every meal, make garlic paste (garlic and cooking oil) in blender, then store in small jars in fridge or freezer to quickly add a spoonful to dishes. A garlic press also works nicely.
- When heating the oven to cook squash, yams, or potatoes, cook more than you will eat and refrigerate for a cold salad, cut and broil for fries, use to thicken soup broth or reheat for another dinner. Cooked and cooled sweet potato and an avocado makes a quick breakfast/lunch.
- Toss favorite vegetables or tofu into marinade while you're working all day. Throw on grill or roast/bake them when you get home.
- In morning, throw broth, legumes, vegetables, spices/salt, onion, and garlic in slow cooker and come home to a cooked meal.

- Leftovers are key! Cook more than you will eat. The next night, just reheat.

Chapter 18
Cost Saving

It is important to debunk some myths running around. More often than I care to hear, people tell me it's too expensive to eat healthy. I personally think it's an excuse that has nothing to stand on. If this is you, all you need to do is decide your health is a priority. And once you do that, your mindset begins to change. This section will give you some great money-saving tips on top of it. I'm here to tell you that you can whip up a delicious healthy meal in 20 minutes without breaking the bank.

Eating healthy on a budget is totally doable! Here's the deal. Yes, organic vegetables and fruit are going to be more expensive than buying conventional produce. But once you realize that there is something terribly amiss when you can get a bushel of strawberries for 99 cents, you best question that produce. I know, I'm exaggerating. I don't even know how much a bushel is but I made a point, right? Same goes for a dozen eggs. Do you really think you are getting healthy eggs at $1-2 a dozen? Seriously? I question the quality of that food. If you pay $4-5 for a dozen eggs, it is still a super cheap meal at less than 40 cents an egg.

It would be nice if you could buy everything organic but that is not always realistic. Until the majority get on board with organic, it may remain pricey. Do what you can to support the organic farms to help lower prices. And always buy organic for the "dirty dozen." The Environmental Working Group (EWG.org), tests produce every year and releases the "dirty dozen" that have the most pesticide residue. Trust me when I say you do not want to be consuming pesticides in great numbers. Some of the common showings on this list tend to be things like apples, strawberries, cherries, peaches, and spinach. It means that not only do these foods have plenty of pesticides sprayed on them, it also means that the food maintains pesticide residue that you ultimately consume. They also list the "Clean 15" which gives you an idea of items that do not use many pesticides and/or don't maintain them inside the food. Some of these items may have thick skin protecting the food inside, like avocados, pineapple, melon, banana and papaya. And items like onions for example don't use much if any pesticides because bugs aren't really attracted to them. Some of this is common sense once you understand the basics.

Let's discuss what doesn't break the bank. Have you been to the bulk aisle recently? I'm not talking about chocolate covered malt balls, I'm talking about dried lentils, beans, and grains like quinoa, rice, black rice, wild rice, millet, amaranth, etc. Not only is this stuff dirt cheap, it will last in the pantry for up to a year. And hold onto your hats people, this is the stuff I literally fuel my body with. Yes, I eat lots and lots of healthy fresh produce, but it's legumes and whole grains chock full of fiber, protein and complex carbohydrates that fills this girl up. Carb is not the dirty word so many think it is especially when it has "complex" before it. Did I mention it's inexpensive?

I'll tell you what IS expensive. Meat and cheese. If you are a fan of animal products, I want to invite you to cut down on it just a bit and choose healthier varieties when you do eat it. I'm talking about grass-fed beef, butter, and cheese as well as poultry that hasn't been injected with hormones and chicken "flavor" before it's wrapped and shipped (seriously, they do that now).

A tad on "grass-fed" beef. The reason why this is so ultra-important is that cows naturally eat grass. They don't go into corn fields and chow down on grain. No, they eat grass, period. But when commercial farms feed the contained cows an unnatural diet of GMO-corn and other fillers, the tissue of the cow no longer has a good balance of omega-3 to omega-6. In fact, it's way loaded on the omega-6 side. And guess what cancer studies tell us? Well, you can probably guess but I'll leave that up to you if you care to research it. But you don't need to do that, do you? All you need to do is look to Mother Nature and ask her. Which basically means, look outside your window when you're driving past a cow pasture and see the cows grazing on grass. (By the way, if you see cows grazing, that would be a sustainable farm, not a conventional one where the cows don't get outside. You won't see those cows). If you're not convinced to cut down on animal products and spend a bit more when you do eat it (on sustainably-raised animals), please do some research—for you and your family's sake.

You know what else is super expensive? Processed foods. Frozen waffles, cereal, crackers, and cookies are expensive, period. And to go a step further, if you add up the nutrition in that food you're getting even less for your money than you thought. Remember, food is to nourish the body. It's not to stuff your stomach so you think you're full for a couple hours only to put strain on your liver for having to process a bunch of chemicals (much of which ends up stored in fat cells). Your body will scream for more food in no time to try to get some amount of nutrition. Save your money and health by avoiding these products.

Please forgive me for ranting. I guess I've bottled up all those excuses I've heard in the past about healthy food being super expensive and only for the elite. It's so not the case and it's time to take responsibility for our health and our eating habits. Keep in mind, the reason you reach for unhealthy processed foods mostly has to do about how you feel about yourself and the stress that overwhelms you. With your 4-Minute Miracle practice, this urge will go way down. So please continue your practice and watch healthier habits come forth.

Also, you don't have to snack on a bunch of expensive super foods to be healthy. There are a lot on the market for those who have the luxury of excess funds. Things like goji berries, mulberries, wheatgrass powder, cultured foods and drinks (which you can make yourself—so easy), raw dehydrated flax crackers, kale chips, and so much more. Most of these have been given the term "super food," but I feel there are plenty of common foods that deserve this title as well. Things like broccoli, cabbage, Brussels sprouts, kale, spirulina, raisins, sweet potatoes, and cranberries, just to name a few. I cannot remember how expensive spirulina is because it lasts forever. I keep mine in the freezer and put 1/2 teaspoon in a smoothie or water. And cranberries may be one of the most undervalued superfoods, which happen to be super easy on the pocketbook. Buy them during Thanksgiving season, keep them in your freezer and throw a handful in your smoothies. They are super cleansing and high in anti-oxidants. You can easily skip the trendy super food aisle if you are watching your budget and stick to more common nutrient-dense foods.

I understand there are many people trying to get by on pennies a day, and it can be challenging to get healthy fresh produce. There are options for you too. I recently heard about "Produce on Wheels" which gives 60 pounds of fresh produce for $10. They come around to about five locations in my area each week to allow people to cash in on this goldmine. Trust me when I say you cannot eat 60 pounds of produce in a week. You can easily share it with at least two other families, which is less than $5 a week. There are other similar organizations as well. Do some research, ask your neighbors and friends to join in. And enjoy your new-found healthy eating lifestyle without breaking the bank.

Chapter 19
Kitchen Staples
and Recipes

Specializing in "practical" whole food preparation allows me to meet you in your busy productive lifestyle. I want to share some of my favorite preparation techniques that keep things healthy, tasty, and practical for the busy person. These plant-based kitchen preparations will also ensure you are filling half your plate with delicious vegetables for optimal cleansing, elimination, dropping excess fat, and alkalizing your meals—a quadruple whammy! If you care to check out some of my plant-based recipe books online, visit the gift shop link at www.TrueBalanceWellness.com.

The very first vegetable preparation that any cooking novice can do is to fill a large CorningWare® type of dish with a bunch of vegetables (whatever floats your boat), drizzle healthy cooking oil, sea salt, and any spices you desire, toss it and throw it in the oven. Feel free to go about doing your laundry, answering email or reading that book while the oven does the leg work. I either cook it at a low temperature like 225 degrees for 90 minutes or so (maintaining much of the nutrients), or if I don't have the luxury of time, I will cook it at a higher heat like 350 degrees for 30 minutes. Depending on the vegetables you use, it will take different cook times. Just poke them with a knife to test when they are tender. These veggies are so delicious with just a little salt and a healthy oil and will pair nicely with any protein or starch.

Slow-Cook Vegetables

<u>Ingredients:</u>

Chopped vegetables of choice
Cooking oil (coconut, avocado)
Sea salt, spice

1. Set oven to 225 -350 degrees F (depending on how much time you have).
2. Chop vegetables of choice (those that will have approximately the same cook time).*
3. Place vegetables in a CorningWare® or oven-safe dish with lid.
4. Toss vegetables with healthy cooking oil (avocado, coconut) and salt, pepper, garlic powder as you wish.
5. Place in oven with lid for 30-90 minutes or until tender. Enjoy.

*General rule of thumb: below-ground root vegetables (potatoes, yams, carrots, radish, turnip, parsnip) will take longer to cook than above-ground (broccoli, cauliflower, eggplant, zucchini, etc.).

If that doesn't knock your socks off, try grilling, steaming (no oil needed), stir-frying (only use quick-cooking veggies), or as I mentioned earlier, my favorite, baking them on a cookie sheet (toss once during cooking). Except for the steaming method, most of these will require some cooking liquid and/or oil. I tend to use a healthy cooking oil, sea salt or tamari (healthier soy sauce), and maybe a splash of vinegar. You will soon find your favorite methods. My cooking oil of choice is coconut or avocado. If cooking on lower temperatures, I will use extra virgin olive oil.

Now, you may not fill up on a meal of vegetables, so I suggest cooking up a grain like quinoa, millet, wild rice or white/black/brown rice along with a good protein like beans, fish or tempeh. Most grains, except for millet, have a 1:2 ratio of grain to cooking liquid (millet 1: 3 1/2). I usually make a big pot of grains, enough for leftovers to use with a soup or stir fry the next night. This will simmer with water on the stove for about 30-40 minutes until all water is absorbed and grains are tender. After cooking has started, avoid stirring your grains, as steam holes will form. If disturbed, your grains may cook unevenly. You can also add some sea salt and coconut oil to your grains and even add a spice blend to get some flavor. I sometimes add a can of vegetable broth or coconut milk (for a savory dish) in place of some water. Add some curry powder and we've got a party, people! Meals like this can be very easy.

Pot of Whole Grains

Ingredients:

1 cup grains/seeds (quinoa, millet, rice, etc.)
2 cups cooking liquid (3 ½ cups for millet)
1/2 teaspoon sea salt
Spices as desired

1. Optional: Soak grains in filtered water for several hours (to make more digestible)
2. Add 1 cup of grains/seeds to pot and add 2 cups cooking liquid (or 3 1/2 cups for millet). Note: cooking liquid can be water, broth, milk (coconut, almond, etc.), lemon/lime juice (counts toward the total liquid content).
3. Add 1/2 teaspoon sea salt and any other spices you desire (garlic powder, pepper, curry, rosemary, etc.)
4. Cover and simmer for cook time for that grain (typically 30-45 minutes).
5. Do not disturb steam holes by stirring until all water is absorbed and grain is tender.
6. Fluff with a fork and enjoy. Refrigerate leftovers up to 4 days.

Note: you can combine grain with vegetables and/or protein in a larger pot for a one-pot meal (see below).

Soups and stews are my all-time favorite—one-pot dishes that you prep and leave alone. Don't reveal whether it is a soup or stew until the dish is done cooking. Sometimes it's hard to gauge how much cooking liquid will be absorbed with all the stuff I'm throwing in there. If it turns out thick, it's a stew. Otherwise it's a soup. Feel free to switch it up for leftovers as you see fit. For example, if it started as a creamy vegetable soup, the next night I may add some rice noodles, lentils or brown rice and make it a thicker dish. I could puree the soup on night two and add some fun toppings like pepitas, pine nuts or spiralized zucchini. Or I may make an acorn squash and spoon the leftovers in it. Seems that leftovers continue to get better during the week as you tweak things. This will come with practice. And as you choose to be present in the kitchen instead of rushing, this intuitive nature reveals itself. If you had told me I would be a savvy cook ten years ago, I would have thought you were crazy. As I mentioned, a bowl of cereal for dinner was commonplace for me then.

I rarely use recipes. When I shop, I buy what is in season, looks fresh, and an amount I think I can use in a week. I always have staples that preserve longer like onions, garlic, celery, carrots and cabbage. Then I supplement with things that look amazingly fresh. I hate to waste any food and find I like the challenge to use everything before it turns. Making soups and stews is a super simple way to throw in a bunch of vegetables you have on hand.

When I am ready to prepare a meal, I go through my garden and fridge and pull together the vegetables of interest. I clean and chop to my heart's content and chop more than I might need for my mystery pot (at this point I have no idea what I am making for dinner yet—stay with me). My very favorite way to cook is to pull out my biggest pot and cutting board and start chopping. My husband often comes through and asks what's for dinner. My common response is, "time will tell."

Since I eat primarily a plant-based diet, I won't be supplementing with any meat so instead I go to the pantry for either a bean, lentil, or whole grain. And if I'm using any starchy vegetables like squash or sweet potatoes, I can forgo the grain or legume as my meal will still be hearty.

I choose a big pot for two people because I then have tomorrow night off. Like I said before, we love leftovers. Sometimes I will freeze half of it for a meal the following week if I want to mix things up.

So here I am with a bowl full of cut-up vegetables and some rinsed legume or grain. It's helpful to heat up the cooking liquid in your pot while you are chopping vegetables to save time. Deciding whether you want to fix a soup, stew or hearty vegetable dish determines the amount of liquid you may need. If you're going for a soup or stew, I might fill the pot with a couple quarts of vegetable broth or just water (if using flavorful veggies) and heat it up. I keep in mind that any grain used will soak up a good amount of liquid.

After the cooking liquid is heated, I throw in all the vegetables, grains or legumes with a generous amount of sea salt and bring to a simmer for 40 minutes or so. I can add spices if I choose. If you are new to the kitchen concept, start easy with oregano for a tomato-ey dish or cumin and coriander for a legume dish. Smell everything before you add it. Or get some spice blends so you don't have to figure out which herbs go well together. Taste after 30 or 40 minutes and adjust your seasoning. Usually you will need more sea salt as I find most people are afraid of it. If you're trying to cut down on salt, a squeeze of lemon will help to naturally bring out the flavor of food and I recommend this anyway. Spicy or smoky herbs like cayenne or smoked paprika are more powerful and will allow you to use less salt as well. If your dish is bland-tasting, you are likely not adding enough salt. And for a flavorful salty addition, tamari can be used as a type of finishing salt. It is a healthier alternative than soy sauce and brings out the flavor of your dish as does salt. The area you should be concerned about sodium consumption is with salty processed or restaurant food. That's where you will run into the most trouble with salt intake.

When the meal is seasoned to my satisfaction, I love to sprinkle on toppings right in the bowls. Try pine nuts or pepitas (pumpkin seeds), cultured veggies (sauerkraut), a drizzle of coconut oil and/or tamari, and some cut-up fresh herbs (parsley, thyme, dill, chives, or cilantro). Feel free to add chopped raw veggies as well like cucumbers, zucchini, or arugula. Toppings are fun and add a bunch of flavor.

Have I lost you yet? Okay, here are the super simple steps I just took to create a pot of wonderful home-cooked goodness.

One-Pot-Meal (template)

<u>Ingredients:</u>

1 cup grains/seeds, lentils, or 3 cups cooked beans, etc.
1-2 quarts cooking liquid
4 cups chopped vegetables (zucchini, broccoli, carrot, celery, onion, garlic, bok choy, cabbage, etc.)
Sea salt and Spices to taste

1. Heat up 1-2 quarts cooking liquid in large pot (broth, water, milk, or other).
2. Chop vegetables—add to pot after liquid is hot (add more liquid if needed to cover vegetables).
3. Add salt, pepper, spices, squeeze of lemon if desired (a splash of cooking oil will help infuse any dry herbs).
4. Simmer 30-40 minutes, taste, adjust spices.
5. Put in bowls, add toppings and enjoy.

Just so I am clear. This is a super-simple process for creating a big pot of nutritious goodness. In culinary school, you might learn that if you sauté the vegetables with oil before adding cooking liquid, your dish will taste better. I use both methods, depending on how I am feeling. Quick cooking lesson… Combining cold water and vegetables is how one makes stock and the vegetables get depleted of flavor (and tossed). You don't want this in your soup which is why I had you heat up the broth before adding the vegetables. If you sauté the vegetables first and toss them with a little oil, however, it will protect the precious veggies from becoming depleted. In this case, you can add cooking liquid hot or cold after sautéing them. I love, love, love, my counter-top water heater that I got for $20 at Costco. I use it all the time to heat water and add to my dishes to speed up cook time.

Remember, when cooking a grain vegetable dish as a one-pot meal, the grain will absorb much liquid. This is okay—unless you want a soup. The vegetables you use will add some water to the dish as well. Be sure to not stir your dish during the grain cooking cycle to maintain the steam holes it creates. After the grain is tender, you can stir the dish and adjust salt and spices. You can also do these slow-cook methods in a crock pot cooking slowly for several hours during the day. Slow cooking on low temperatures maintains much nutrition in your food.

If you are not kitchen-savvy, don't get overwhelmed. Commit to learning something new every week. You will be amazed at how quickly it all comes together with a little practice.

Use the recipe template above for a general one-pot meal or follow one of my favorite one-pot meal recipes below to get you started:

Coconut Curry Millet and Vegetables

Can make the grain in separate pan or throw all together in one for easy one-pot meal.

Ingredients:

Veggies:	2 small zucchinis, 1 small onion, 4 garlic cloves, minced
Veggies:	½ cup peas and/or green beans, 1 can water chestnuts
Grain:	½ cup millet, soaked 2-8 hrs, rinse well
Herb/spice	1 t sea salt, 1 t garlic powder, 2 t curry powder
Cooking liquid:	1 can coconut milk, plus ¾ cup water

1. Seal first set of vegetables with a bit of coconut oil in frying pan on medium heat. Let cook for 5 minutes, stirring a couple times.
2. Add rinsed grain, cooking liquid (milk and water), and rest of vegetables, along with salt, herbs/spices.
3. Bring to boil, turn down heat to low and simmer for 30-45 minutes or until water is absorbed.

Smokey White Bean Soup

When thinking about using white beans in a soup, I automatically saw carrots and curly kale in it to offset the "white" in the beans, creating a soup appealing to the eye.

Ingredients:

2 cups curly kale, spinach, or chard chopped small (or 1 cup parsley)
1 medium onion, chopped
4-5 garlic cloves, minced
3 stalks celery, chopped
3 carrots, chopped
3 cups cooked white beans
1-2 cups coconut milk plus enough water to cover beans by two inches
2 T lemon juice or splash of balsamic vinegar

Sea salt and pepper to fit
1-inch ginger root, grated
2 t garlic powder
2 bay leaves
1 chili pepper (without seeds)
~30 drops liquid smoke (optional)
3 T tamari finishing salt (if needed)

1. Sauté onion for 5 minutes. Chop rest of veggies (except leafy greens i.e. kale) and seal one at a time (celery, carrot) with a bit of coconut oil. This step will seal the vegetables to maintain their integrity.
2. Add cooking liquid (milk, water, lemon), cooked beans, and all herb/spice including salt & pepper and allow to heat and cook for 20 minutes. Add chopped leafy greens.
3. Taste for salt. Adjust seasoning and allow to cook another 10 minutes. Repeat until veggies are tender and broth is tasty. Add finishing salt—tamari if needed. Full cooking time may be 45min – 1 hr.
4. Top soup bowls with avocado and fresh herbs. Enjoy.

Note: You may also try to throw everything in a crock pot and cook all day on low. If using dried beans, soak overnight first, rinse, then add ingredients to crock pot and cook all day.

Rice Noodle Vegetable Soup

Similar to the popular PHO soup, this soup is super simple - throw everything together in a pot. Pull out any and all vegetables you may have in the fridge and go to town. This recipe will show you my favorite veggies to add, but most any veggie will work. A simple vegetable soup can be raised to fabulous with some creative toppings like fresh herbs, pumpkin seeds, drizzling coconut oil for creaminess, dried seaweed strips and/or cultured vegetables.

Ingredients:

1-quart vegetable broth (plus more hot water as needed)
1 onion (red or yellow)
3-4 garlic cloves (or 1 T garlic mash)
4-5 cups vegetables (2 carrots, 1 zucchini, ½ C snow peas, 1 small can sliced water chestnuts, 2 C chopped green cabbage, 1 C mushrooms)
2 handfuls rice noodles
Salt/pepper to taste
Garnish ideas: fresh basil or cilantro, pumpkin seeds, drizzle coconut oil, seaweed strips, cultured vegetables
Optional: 1 T miso paste per bowl

1. Heat broth on stove to simmer as you chop vegetables (carrots can be shredded for quicker soup).
2. Add vegetables to hot broth and bring back to simmer. Add noodles and simmer for 20 minutes.
3. Garnish with fresh basil or cilantro, pumpkin seeds, seaweed strips, coconut oil.

Optional: for probiotic activity and extra flavor, add 1 T miso paste to bowl with some of the broth. Whisk until mixed in, add more soup. Enjoy.

Wild Rice Sweet Potato Stew

Super hearty and delicious. Wild rice is a grass, not a grain. Switch up your usual grains for nutrition variety. This dish is nice in a crock pot cooking all day. Ensure you have enough liquid as the wild rice will soak up at least two cups of liquid.

Ingredients:

1 jar diced tomatoes
1-quart vegetable broth plus hot water to cover by 2 in.
1 onion (red or yellow)
3-4 garlic cloves (or 1 T premade garlic oil – see time saving tips)
4-5 cups vegetables (2 carrots, 2 stalks celery, 1 zucchini, 4 red potatoes, 2-4 red sweet potatoes or yams)
1 cup wild rice, rinsed and soaked for 8+ hours
Salt/pepper/garlic powder to taste
Garnish: drizzle coconut oil, cultured vegetables

1. Rinse and soak wild rice for 8+ hours. This will allow the rice to cook more quickly and digest more easily. If you don't have time for this step, you may want to boil the rice before adding it to your dish.
2. Heat broth on stove to simmer as you chop vegetables.
3. Add vegetables, garlic, salt, pepper to hot broth and bring back to simmer.
4. Add wild rice and simmer 45 minutes.

5. Taste and add seasoning/tamari (finishing salt) as necessary.
6. Garnish as desired. Enjoy.

Breakfast time seems to be challenging for many because most want something hearty to stay satisfied, yet want it to be super simple. I always seem to enjoy my morning smoothie where I can throw in a bunch of essential nutrition to get the day started right. See below for what I put in my smoothies. If adding protein powder, I prefer plant-based with either sprouted or fermented grains for easier assimilation. Many protein powders today are hard to digest and hard on the intestinal walls.

Another morning ritual began several years ago when I discovered chia porridge. It's healthier than oatmeal (up for debate), packs more protein, and literally takes 4 minutes to prepare. You basically add chia seeds to a bowl, warm water, and any toppings you desire. Let it thicken for two minutes and you've got a bowl of wholesome deliciousness. You could also prepare it the night before and allow it to thicken in a Mason jar in the fridge. Be sure to have plenty of liquid so the chia does not form a thick ball, which could be harder to digest. Oats can also be consumed raw if they are soaked overnight or soaked in hot water for 10 minutes.

Chia Porridge

Ingredients:

Liquid:	¾ C fresh nut milk or water (warm will thicken more quickly)
Protein:	4 T whole or ground chia seeds
Flavor:	sliced fruit, berries, etc.
Sweet:	as desired - 4 drops stevia OR ½ T pure maple syrup or honey
Other Ideas:	Splash of nut milk, chopped nuts/seeds, cinnamon, coconut flakes, cacao powder

1. Mix chia seeds and warm water in a bowl. Add rest of desired ingredients as chia thickens (2-4min with warm water, more with cold). Stir and enjoy.

Power Smoothie

Mix up this nutrient-rich smoothie in a blender until smooth. Adjust liquid content as desired.

Ingredients:

Liquid: 1 cup fresh water (add 4-5 almonds for almond milk)
Vitamins: 2 large handfuls of greens
(romaine, kale, chard, beet greens, spinach)
Acid/cuts bitter: ¼ lemon
Fatty Acids: 1-2 T seeds (chia, flax, hemp)

Liver Health: 1-2 t milk thistle seeds
Anti-oxidants: 1 C frozen berries
Anti-inflammatory: 1 t turmeric spice
Nutrition Powerhouse: 1 t moringa powder
Protein: 1 scoop plant protein

How about a super simple blender soup for lunch? In fact, if you're a smoothie maniac and use your blender every morning, simply rinse it out and prep your lunch before fully washing the blender. Store it in the fridge in a Mason jar until lunchtime. You may already have guessed it but if you don't have any Mason jars, you might want to start saving glass jars with lids. This is an easy way to transport your lunch to work as needed and keeps things fresh in the fridge. And if you have a quick water heater like I do, you can substitute hot water for a warm soup in just minutes.

Quick Chilled Blender Soup

Ingredients:

Liquid: 1-2 cups cold water
Fat: 2 t olive oil, 1/8 C tahini
Veggies: 2 stalks celery, 1 red pepper, 1 tomato, ½ cucumber, ¼ c onion
Herbs/Spice: ¼ cup cilantro,1 clove garlic, 2 T lemon, small jalapeno (seeded)
Salt: 1 t sea salt, ¼ t miso paste (optional)
Sweet: 1 apple
Topping: chopped avocado and/or pine nuts

127

1. Put all ingredients into blender and blend until still slightly chunky or to desired consistency.
2. Put in bowl and enjoy! Add toppings if desired.

Since we're on the blender topic, I'd like to share one of my all-time favorite patés. They are so easy and delicious with just a few ingredients. It's kind of like hummus (recipe below), but using nuts instead of beans. The store-bought hummus today is disappointing me more and more with unhealthy oils and even water added, which makes it go rancid quickly. Try a paté substitute for hummus to spice up your routine.

Walnut Paté

Ingredients:

2 cups of walnuts
1 stalk celery
½ red bell pepper
2 green onions
½ t sea salt (or to taste)

1. Soak nuts in water overnight (or 4 hours) and rinse well. This step is optional but helps digestibility of the nuts.
2. Process all ingredients in food processor until smooth.
3. Great on top of sliced red bell peppers, carrots, crackers, etc.

Hummus

Ingredients:

1, 15-oz can of chickpeas (garbanzo beans)
1 clove garlic, plus 1 t garlic powder
1 jalapeno pepper, seeded, chopped (optional)
¼ C tahini and/or olive oil
2 T + fresh lemon juice
1 t ground cumin
Sea salt to taste (~1/2 t)
½ C fresh cilantro (or other fresh herbs)
Pepitas and/or smoked paprika (for garnish)

1. Rinse beans well under cool water.
2. Put all ingredients (except herbs and pepitas) in food processor or blender and blend until creamy. Add more oil and/or lemon to thin as needed. Taste for salt. Adjust as needed.
3. Add fresh herbs and pulse a few times to blend in.
4. Put in bowl and garnish with pepitas and smoked paprika.
5. Serve with veggies, on romaine leaves, or roll into a chard leaf.

It is also important to have some treats on hand for when your sweet tooth makes itself known. It's amazing how scrumptious healthy desserts can be. I like to make bars with cacao powder (raw cocoa powder), some type of fruit to sweeten them, like dates, raisins, or figs, and nuts and/or seeds to add some savory fat. First, process the nuts to a powder, maybe adding some oil to create a nut-butter consistency. Add pitted dates (soaked if too dry) or raisins and any flavorings like cacao powder, cinnamon, nutmeg, etc. Process it all together and taste. If it needs sweetness, add some. If it needs to be smoother, add some oil, nut butter, or pumpkin puree—get creative. Add some texture with seeds, chopped nuts, or coconut flakes. Either roll into bite-sized balls or press the mixture into a loaf or cake pan and refrigerate until hardened. You can then slice small bites and put them in the freezer so you don't eat them all in one sitting. They are that good! You can pull one out of the freezer anytime you need to satisfy your sweet tooth naturally, or you need a quick breakfast as you rush out the door. It's essential to have this on hand to avoid the cookie jar or whatever your nemesis might be. Here is a recipe to get you started:

Date/Nut Bars

Ingredients:

1 ½ cup nuts (cashews, almonds or walnuts or ¾ C nut butter
¼ C tahini (or almond butter)
6 pitted dates (1/2 C)
1 ½ t vanilla extract (or ½ t vanilla powder)
¼ t sea salt
¼ C hemp hearts and/or sesame seeds
2 T cacao powder

1. If dates are dry and hard, soak for 20 minutes or so.
2. Put 1 ½ cup nuts in food processor and process until powdery.
3. Add rest of ingredients and process. Taste and adjust as needed.
4. Press into small loaf pan (or roll into balls). Add garnish if desired (hemp hearts, sesame, etc.)
5. Place in fridge for 1 hour or overnight. Cut up and freeze for quick bites.

I have dabbled in other sweet treats over the years that are still quite healthy such as my black bean brownies, lemon scones, or pumpkin bread. I have figured out a way to bake without refined grains or sugar. I will go more into these items in book 2 on gut health.

Salad dressing is another super simple staple and will cut down on unhealthy store-bought varieties that use cheap oils. You will start to save *mucho dollares* when you stop buying that expensive processed stuff. In many cases I like to simply add olive oil, vinegar, and either coconut aminos or sea salt to a salad. Augmenting the oil and vinegar with something salty like aminos or tamari adds so much to the dressing and brings out some amazing flavors in your veggies. Here is a simple recipe with some options for thicker creamier dressings:

Salad Dressing

Ingredients:

1 C Fat: (olive oil, avocado oil, and/or tahini/nut butter)
1/4 C Acid: lemon juice or vinegar (coconut, apple cider, balsamic)
½ t Salt: (sea salt, aminos, or miso paste)

Optional:

Thickener: (½ avocado, 2 T miso paste, mustard, tahini, or nut butter)
Thin: (water, lemon juice, oil, etc.)
Flavor: (herbs, garlic, onion, sesame oil, tamari, sea salt)

1. Mix all ingredients using an emersion blender, whisk, blender or fork. Store in Mason jar.

In addition to salads, I also sprinkle the dressing on top of steamed or baked veggies and grain dishes if they are lacking pizazz. You can add any flavoring by way of spices or even fruits. You can thicken your dressings with a spoonful of mustard, miso paste, avocado, or some blended cashews. Sometimes I put tomato and basil in a blender with oil, vinegar and sea salt for a delicious change of pace on my salad. Use healthy oils such as organic cold pressed extra virgin olive oil. Dressings are fun to create but in a pinch, remember, it's as easy as oil, vinegar, and sea salt/aminos. Coconut vinegar is a mild vinegar with a hint of sweetness and is my favorite. I enjoy balsamic vinegar, too, but do not use it often due to the sulfites added.

Speaking of salads, the easiest way to spruce one up without chopping a bunch of vegetables is spooning some cultured veggies onto your greens to add a quick punch of nutrition and color. I then like to add avocado, Kalamata olives, and nuts or seeds for some extra protein and heartiness. It's not uncommon for me to add beans, lentils, or leftover grains as well. If you need to make your salad sustain you until dinner, it is a must.

For a quick hearty protein lunch in a hurry, open a can of garbanzo beans, also known as chickpeas, rinse them well, and sprinkle with some oil, vinegar, and sea salt or coconut aminos. If you want to get more creative, cut up fresh herbs, avocado, and add seeds for a crunch. And feel free to add these beans to a prepared greens salad for extra protein. As an added tip, if you smash the beans with a fork, they will absorb more of the dressing/seasoning.

Another quick hearty lunch is cut-up leftover (cooked) sweet potato, avocado sprinkled with coconut aminos (or sea salt), and pepitas. You've got yourself a winner here. Super simple, savory and satisfying.

As you start to learn some of these staples, you will immediately gain access to your natural creative juices. You have an instinct to create healthy natural foods from the earth. Your taste buds will guide you. Don't feel overwhelmed and don't throw out all the old stuff just yet. Tackle one thing at a time. Baby steps. You can handle this one moment, this one task. You can do this.

You may not like being in the kitchen now, but don't underestimate the power of this work and the changes in front of you. I never thought I would enjoy being in the kitchen. I was the one eating cereal for dinner every night after a hard day in the corporate madness, remember? And when I did prepare a meal, I was too focused on the result and not enjoying the process. Learn from my mistakes. Be with the food, appreciate it fully, and you will find that you prefer spending extra time in the kitchen rather than catching that sitcom later.

There is time for sitcoms, but your priorities will shift and suddenly there is plenty of time and energy to prepare healthy meals. You have more energy when it doesn't feel like a task. It becomes a time of presence and rejuvenation for your spirit. And once you see how food can transform your health, you will love being in the kitchen and sharing healthy food with others. Trust me for now, until you can experience it for yourself. And find more recipes on my blog at www.TrueBalanceWellness.com or purchase my plant-based recipe e-books in the gift shop.

Section Review

- Clean up your kitchen and purchase any necessary tools to make your time efficient.
- Prepare for presence in the kitchen and see your energy reserves replenish.
- Decide that your health is important and commit to your kitchen time.
- Refer to the chapter on time-saving tips to keep your time in the kitchen concise, enjoyable, affordable, and practical.
- Go to EWG.com for the latest data on which foods to buy organic ("dirty dozen") and which can be conventional ("clean 15").
- Shop the bulk aisle for dry grains, legumes, nuts and seeds.
- Choose sustainably-raised animal products and eat them less often if you need to reduce your grocery bill (replace with legumes and other high-quality plant protein).
- Cut back on processed foods to save on your grocery bill and chose whole foods for the biggest bang for your buck.
- Check out low-cost local food options like "produce on wheels" or "bountiful baskets" or food banks.
- Refer to the Kitchen Staples chapter for a quick start to easy meals and filling half your plate with fat-crushing alkalizing vegetables. And check out my plant-based recipe books on the "gift shop" link at www.TrueBalanceWellness.com

Part 6:
Solidifying Your Sexy

Chapter 20
Commit to You

Hopefully you have implemented The 4-Minute Miracle and are on your way to revealing your sexy. Are you seeing the benefits from this practice yet? Or did you discount it because you think it is too simple or downright silly? Whether or not you've begun your practice, can I ask you to trust me and this process for a bit longer?

You'll see that with this practice, punishing your body will soon be a thing of the past. Your primary reason to eat will be to nourish the body as opposed to disrespecting and sabotaging it. Simply put, your body doesn't deserve that punishment. Instead, you will eat more slowly and deliberately, you will eat less, and likely gravitate toward real food, i.e., healthier food for your body. And I'm telling you this comes naturally after implementing The 4-Minute Miracle—almost without effort. When you connect with you, the emotions around food soften and stress-eating diminishes.

The other concepts in this book are extremely helpful, but this is where we finally win this food war. This is the true gem. If you have kids, there is nothing greater you can do for them than committing to yourself first. When you do so, they believe it's okay to treat themselves well. Do you want your kids to have a good relationship with food and with themselves? Of course you do. Your kids don't need *your* love and approval as much as they need their own love and approval. Think about that for a minute and decide if you truly believe it.

This ritual is not time-consuming but is a commitment with results that greatly outweigh the effort. And that is an understatement. I'm going to go out on a limb and say *you have to do this*. It is the only logical choice. If you are reading these words, it's time for you to wake up to the glory your life can be. I *gently* invite you to join me in making this practice a daily ritual in your life today.

Your life will soon be incomplete without this practice. We are taught to fast forward through the pauses in life. But now I *want* you to pause ... for four minutes each and every day.

And during this practice I want you to take the time to acknowledge the person inside that you've likely shoved in the corner while you were making waves in the world. I'm not even asking you to stop making waves. I'm sure you are a great wave-maker. Continue to do your stuff but pause once during your day for the new you.

Is it really that easy, you ask? Yes. Showing up IS easy and that is all I am asking. What comes from showing up is acknowledgment of you. But you must show up. It's really the only hurdle to get over before you start to see the benefits. Is your life worth this commitment for your health and vitality? How about for revealing your sexy?

This book does not suggest a daily meditation practice although if that is your cup of tea, I encourage you to continue to do so. It will pair nicely with this practice. Some people are great meditators. Not me. And I suspect not many of you. Shutting the mind off sounds like a piece of cake but for whatever reason, as soon as I close my eyes and attempt to be quiet, my ego thinks I have created a platform for her as she starts rambling on like a drunk sailor. I don't want to knock meditation. I still attempt it on a pretty regular basis. And when I am able to tap into that space between the thoughts, that place of bliss, I am taken to another dimension. It is heavenly.

But I find there are other ways to tap into this space that are not only easier, they also address an area often missed with meditation. You don't even have to close your eyes (and I suggest you don't). And once you utilize this simple tool for tapping into the real you, meditation will become easier if you choose to go there.

The practice described in this book gives you a focal point, namely *you,* that not only allows you to get acquainted with yourself, but also shuts the ego down for a bit. It becomes much easier to keep the mind quiet during the blissful four minutes.

The 4-Minute Miracle is a method of connecting with your Inner Self, that self we cram down with food, busyness, and nonsense. We tend to ignore the Child Within who is looking for connection, looking for comfort. How did we lose this connection and forget about her? How did we move from this happy-go-lucky child to a serious workaholic who stuffs meals down like she's in the middle of a marathon? It's in this chaos that we lost our way. We lost ourselves in the subconscious eating frenzy that is all too common for most. It's time to take a moment, literally four minutes, to reconnect and regain our composure internally and reflect that outward into the world.

The place where you will find comfort is in stopping and acknowledging. When you stop for four minutes a day, something miraculous happens. Everything halts and you can see clearly. And guess what? This connection transfers to the dinner table. You may no longer feel anxious throughout the day when you take these four minutes committed to simply acknowledging yourself. When you implement The 4-Minute Miracle, you may notice a world of change happening inside and out. Take notice.

Today I find it hard to get through a whole day without this quiet time where I acknowledge myself. It calms me. It clarifies my purpose and passion. Without purpose, it is easy to turn to food or some other vice to try to fill a void. But all becomes quiet and clear when I connect with the self. This practice allows me to connect with my heart as my ego quietly stays in the background. This quiet time is a ritual I respect and honor now. And my child-self certainly deserves this commitment to her.

With a type-A personality and a perfectionist streak to boot, it was challenging for me to establish this ritual. I knew how good it felt to go there and yet I would continue to knock things off the to-do list, trying to create artificial value in my life. My advice—establish a ritual as soon as you can that you do no matter what. Pull out every ounce of determination to give this a go. Don't wait as I did. Establish a reward system for doing your practice – whatever it takes.

Chapter 21
Transparency

The 4-Minute Miracle is going to bring more transparency into your life. Let's discuss transparency for a moment. Those living under the same roof likely know you better than you know yourself (unless you're already well on your way with The 4-Minute Miracle). Whether you like it or not, you are already transparent with others – and unfortunately that includes not only your amazing qualities, but also your flaws, insecurities, and worries. It is only yourself you are truly hiding from.

Have you ever noticed someone who just doesn't feel comfortable looking into your eyes while talking to them? You can sense their discomfort as they try to hide a part of themselves. But it's not hidden at all, is it? Nope. It's out there for all to see. And likely you do it too when feeling insecure.

People walk around with humped shoulders, displaying a broken heart they are trying to protect, or crossed arms, displaying frustration. Body language shows us a lot. If you don't think others see your insecurities and emotion, you're mistaken. They may not understand what specific experience caused it, but they can see it exists. Your insecurities limit you and your relationships. This is no way to live. You are blocking all creative expression and authenticity for the life you were meant to live. It's time to take back your power.

If you don't care what others think of you, good for you. But you may want to consider living your best authentic life possible and feeling great as a bonus. And that may require looking at yourself so you can show up in the world with all of your beautiful attributes shining. That's when your mojo comes through, and where you feel amazing to be alive. Do you ever recognize others who are deeply attractive even though their "looks" are just average? It is likely their confidence and healthy self-esteem that attracts you. You can radiate that, too.

I invite you to be voluntarily transparent in the world with your wonderful attributes as well as your flaws. Yes, I said flaws. Put them out there for the world to see. Hate to break it to you, but you're not the only one with flaws and those flaws are likely not all that unique. Others will appreciate your authenticity because they can relate. And remember, they see them anyway.

Let's take an exaggerated example to demonstrate transparency. There is nothing less attractive than someone getting caught in a lie and continuing to deny it. This happens all the time with politicians. They will even go on camera denying something until they're blue in the face while Americans sit back and shake their heads. If, on the other hand, they just took ownership and showed some remorse or compassion, they would come out on top. I can think of a small handful of well-known people who have taken this road. We can find compassion for them when they take responsibility. They are human after all and humans make mistakes. But it's the truly authentic ones that take responsibility.

Even though you may not be on camera, you are transparent, too. Transparency and authenticity can only be achieved if you are first transparent with yourself. Don't worry, it sounds scary until you get comfortable with The 4-Minute Miracle. Soon enough you will agree that you're not all that bad and you can show up completely as you.

Let's go a bit deeper with this concept. Have you ever come across a friend who suddenly became super vulnerable in some manner? Perhaps her partner left her or she got a devastating health diagnosis. Regardless of the circumstance, her heart is exposed and raw and we seem to melt into it. She is real, she is human, she feels, and she is sharing these raw emotions with no one other than you. You feel honored and close to this person in that moment as your heart opens and expands. This is where true heart connections occur—in the moment of vulnerability and transparency. And it's in these moments that our relationships become real. These heart-felt connections do not happen when we are trying to impress someone with our new business suit and freshly painted lipstick. Think about it. Start to observe what you are attracted to and then decide how you want to show up.

You may also experience this closeness with someone you've never met perhaps a reality TV contestant showing vulnerability. Now, I'm not telling you to go out to the grocery store and tell every person you bump into about how you were emotionally or physically abused by your ex, for example. But what I am saying is that you can stop hiding aspects of yourself and watch your true authenticity surface. To do this in the outside world, you first need to simply face yourself. Acknowledge the person inside of you. The rest comes naturally.

Chapter 22
Presence is Key

I keenly recognize what it is like to not know oneself. As I look back over my life it is clear to me that I tried to please others most of my life. I really wasn't even living for me. Or perhaps the "love" I thought I was getting in return was what I longed for.

I now have deep love and respect for myself, or at least a good strong glimpse of it. I know deep in my core how essential it is for contentment and fulfillment in my life. Relationships with anyone else are not truly authentic without first knowing and accepting myself. The 4-Minute Miracle is the secret weapon in my heart-felt opinion, experience, and wisdom. And the best part is that it's super easy to do.

Today I feel genuine—genuinely me with whomever I come across, be it my partner, mother, cat, or neighbor. When I can look at myself in the mirror, literally and figuratively, I can go about my day with grace and ease. Today I often hear people tell me how ravishing I look or that something is different about me. I'm no supermodel, trust me. With this work, something energetic and magical happens. You might describe it in another as poise, grace, or ease. It has to do with a good self-image which leads to confidence and ease with life. And isn't that where feeling sexy comes from? Sure, you may implement techniques in this book that cause excess weight to drop off allowing you to fit into that cocktail dress, but it's really the internal sexy that matters most.

Do you want to solidify the relationship you have with yourself? The 4-Minute Miracle works to acknowledge the self to transform your relationship with food. You may notice that your practice works on other levels as well. Perhaps you notice your ability to speak up for yourself and make better choices. Clarity comes from this practice. You may notice not only the relationship with yourself blossoming but with others as well. It may stop the stress-eating binges, but it also may stop you from blaming others for your circumstances. This is because the clarity we feel and see settles our fears and relaxes them. You may notice life nudging you into more purposeful activities and connections. And hopefully with a better relationship with food, you notice physical changes begin to take form.

One of the important aspects of this practice is presence. This is a key ingredient to shifting your life. All that is required of you is to show up and be present with whatever is in front of you, including the person in your mirror. That is truly all that is required at any moment. And if you are truly present, transparency and authenticity result. And miracles follow.

Most of us, myself included, have lots to do and move quickly through our productive days with intention and efficiency. I used to honor this. Today I contemplate it. I start to question all I *need* and *want* to do. Why do I want all these accomplishments? Do I think they will give me value or happiness somehow? The finish line is where the happiness appears, right? Does the finish line ever appear? Every morning I wake with another task list for another go. And of course, frustration peaks when things get in the way of my productivity.

And so I take a breath and I remind myself that happiness is in each moment, not in the results of circumstances or actions. And so I ask myself, am I happy? Right now? Right in the middle of one of my *worthy* tasks?

It is in those moments of frustration that life is telling me to slow down and become present. This allows me to become open to life. Each single solitary moment is true bliss if you allow it. Each moment has the opportunity for a peaceful experience—even mourning a loved one. If you settle into yourself and the moment, you can find the bliss, the stillness, the answers, the clarity, within it – deep within it. And so, I choose to be still, to be present for all of life. Each moment, each word, each glance, each touch, each tear. Today I choose presence.

Will I feel like I am not intelligent or valued if my agenda stops driving the show? You see, this is the secret to a happy life, where our sexy emerges. The secret is in letting go of whatever you are holding so tightly. It is in the letting go and letting life take the wheel.

Picture yourself rowing upstream to get to your destination and goals only to run into obstacles and fatiguing yourself in the process. Instead of continuing this madness, close your eyes and let go of the oars.

Feel the boat turn and steady itself into the stream of the flowing river. You are now on a ride—one that you no longer direct or control. Your agendas are gone and you can flow freely enjoying the breeze on your skin and the environment around you. The water feels alive as it takes you on a glorious ride, running swiftly and gracefully through the currents. You are delighted in the journey itself and care not where you are headed. As you relax more fully, the journey slows down as you rest and renew and take in its beauty.

Isn't that a beautiful representation of letting go of the wheel we have gripped so tightly? Jerry and Esther Hicks put this vision into my head from one of their talks. Whenever I find myself struggling, I visualize myself in that canoe, letting go of the oars once again.

Letting go allows life to show you the way. Your job is simply to be present and enjoy the experiences life brings you. You win when you can appreciate and allow life to show up for you. This is where your life can take great form. With ease and grace comes a life of fulfilling triumphs one moment at a time, at just the right time. It is in this place that your answers surface. Just showing up with presence allows life to flow rhythmically around you. Isn't this what we all want? Just show up.

Just to be clear, I am not telling you to stop taking steps and putting action to your goals. But when you pause through life, you get more clarity on which direction is most purposeful for you. And in each action, presence is the key.

I invite you to consciously incorporate presence into your life wherever you are. And The 4-Minute Miracle practice will help solidify it. Whenever you find yourself forcing the wheel of your life one way or another, simply become conscious of it and ease up. Yield to life.

Chapter 23
Your Practice

Whether you implemented The 4-Minute Miracle days, weeks, hours ago, or if you are choosing to do so now, we will recap those steps here and give you some additional statements for your Inner Child as she may be ready to hear more from you. Feel free to diverge from these statements as you sense what she needs to hear. If you look deep enough, and feel deep enough, and get your ego out of the way, the right words will reveal themselves. And you may not even need words at all. You are connected to this child and simply feeling the appreciation for her may seal this bond for you. Do not feel you need to follow my instructions. These are simply here to get you started on nurturing that Child Within and acknowledging him or her.

With my own practice, I enjoy journaling after The 4-Minute Miracle, as it often reveals deeper messages for me. Perhaps this early message from my Inner Child may help you understand yours.

As I sit and be with you today I see something deep inside. I sense there is something lying beneath the surface ever so gently stirring and wondering if I will acknowledge it. It is softly calling to me. "I am here. I am

*waiting here for you to see me. It's all I want from you,"
she says. "I feel seen from you, yet I'm cautiously
standing by, still afraid to come forth. Can you just sit
with me today? It feels comforting to know you will take
the time to sit with me and stop running your busy life that
screams your name all day. I feel honored you are with
me, if only for a moment. Thank you for acknowledging
me. Thank you for seeing me. Thank you."*

I hope you honor your self-commitment practice as
I do. If you stick with it, I promise you will see results.
Trust me and stick with it. You are on your way to
revealing your sexy and so much more.

If you are clear on your "why," you can easily get
your sexy back with four minutes dedicated to none
other than you. These four minutes bring clarity, peace,
and acceptance as you bond with your Inner Child who
has been waiting for you. Go to her with compassion
and acceptance, which all children desire and deserve.
You deserve this.

Are you willing to commit to a practice for your
well-being for a mere four minutes each day? Don't let
this miracle slip by you. It's simple but mighty. Take
the leap and join me on this journey.

The 4-Minute Miracle Instructions
(for revealing your sexy):

Find a special place where you can easily sit in front of
a mirror, feet flat on the floor (or lotus position). For the
first few days you may want to just sit and look in your
eyes. After you get comfortable just sitting with yourself,

pick one or two statements below and slowly and deliberately say them into your eyes. See how it feels to you. If something else comes up, speak freely to her. What does your Inner Child need to hear on this day? What does she need to hear to know you are there for her? Sitting with her may be all she needs right now. Acknowledge her. Do feelings and emotions come up? Be with those feelings. Feel them fully and have compassion for them. Here are some compassionate words I might say to my Inner Child to acknowledge her:

- There is no place I would rather be than here with you, right now.
- This is the most important thing I will do all day.
- You are safe.
- There are no expectations here. There is no one to please. We can just be.
- I can simply be me. I am enough.
- This place, right here, right now, feels heavenly.
- Thank you for taking the time to be here with me.
- I feel so blessed to be you/me (whichever word feels better to you).
- Thank you for being you.
- I am committed to you.
- I am here for you today.
- I feel blessed to have found you again.
- Thank you for being with me today.
- Do you need anything from me? I am here for you.

Next Steps

When you are ready to go deeper into this practice, please pick up book two in the series, The 4-Minute Miracle and Gut Health. In this book, we will take a deep dive into one of the best kept anti-aging secrets ever. We are going to transform health and vitality from the inside out. Whether you have a life-limiting diagnosis, or you simply want to slow the aging process, we must focus on one of the least appreciated yet most impactful systems for overall health. This book will reveal and supply simple step-by-step instructions to clean, hydrate, and nourish the gut for long-term health and vitality. Your well-being may dramatically change after implementing these protocols. And finally, this book will go deeper into The 4-Minute Miracle to move from acknowledgement to acceptance of your Inner Child as you build confidence, allowing your sexy to solidify even more. It is in this place that people will wonder about the secret to the sparkle that envelops your essence. I hope to meet you there.

And if you care to dive further into the act of presence and purpose, please find my first book Pebbles of Gold: Finding Inner Nirvana Amidst the Chaos of Life on Amazon or at PebblesofGold.com.

And finally, please check in with me to share your journey with a trusted community. Find me at <u>TrueBalanceWellness.com</u>, <u>LindaCurry.com</u>, and on social media channels.

The 4-Minute Miracle Book Highlights

- Start your 4-Minute Miracle practice and watch your emotions around food settle down.
- Determine your *"why"* for wanting health and vitality. Go deep.
- Slash depriving yourself and feelings of guilt after indulging. Instead *allow* yourself pleasure enjoying every morsel.
- Continue your 4-minute ritual to bring acknowledgment to your Child Within.
- Stop dieting and create healthy habits instead based on your individual needs. Take it one step at a time and start to substitute healthier options.
- Create food rules that tailor to your lifestyle and challenge areas to put willpower (constant food decisions) aside.
- How active would you like to be when you are 80 years old? Do those things today.
- Consider a new love affair with the all-mighty vegetable, assuring plenty of color for an array of nutrition. Try different cooking methods to find your favorites.

- Eat real food that comes from the earth. Boxed food just isn't fuel for the body and is likely zapping your vitality little by little.

- Create a meal plan the night before to avoid willpower coming into play when you are hungry and stressed.

- Consider intermittent fasting to allow the body to continue healing and rejuvenating after sleep.

- Clean up your kitchen and plan to purchase tools to make your time efficient.

- Prepare for presence in the kitchen and see your energy reserves replenish.

- Decide that your health is important and commit to your kitchen time.

- Refer to the time-saving chapter for tips to keep your time in the kitchen concise, enjoyable, affordable, and practical.

- Go to EWG.com for the latest data on which foods to buy organic ("dirty dozen") and which can be conventional ("clean 15").

- Shop the bulk isle for dry grains, legumes, nuts and seeds.

- Choose sustainably-raised animal products and eat less often if you need to reduce your grocery bill.

- Cut back on processed foods to save on your grocery bill and chose whole foods for the biggest bang for your buck.

- Check out low cost local food options like "produce on wheels" or "bountiful baskets" or food banks.

- Refer to the Kitchen Staples chapter for a quick start to easy meals and filling half your plate with fat-crushing alkalizing vegetables.
- See more plant-based recipes on my blog or in the gift shop at <u>www.TrueBalanceWellness.com</u>
- Consider transparency and authenticity in your life.
- Continue The 4-Minute Miracle practice daily to calm the stress and eating triggers in your life and revealing that sexy within.

Acknowledgments

Other than my mother who engrained good eating and taking care of myself from a very young age, there are many people who supported the process of bringing <u>The 4-Minute Miracle</u> to life. Tom Bird and his team, Sabrina and John, thank you for your gentle guidance and inspiration. The 4-Minute Miracle focus group participants, thank you for your honest, raw feedback from your experiences. To my reviewers who gave encouraging yet constructive critiques to better guide the final manuscript: Valerie, Alistair, Jessica, Evelyn, Claire, Barbara, Karla, Carolyn, Christy, Nicole, Marie – thank you. A special and grateful shout-out to my line editor Charlotte Dixon and final editor, Beth Livengood. My Mesa writing support team encouraging me every step of the way: Jessica, Claire, Wendy, Sheryl and Lori. And my online writer support team who joined our virtual writing sessions and offered needed encouragement: David, Jessica, Evelyn, Yvonne, Angie, Nancy, Monica, Jane.

Finally, my husband Rich. You continue to cheer on my love of writing and giving back to the world. Your support is beyond words. You've given me the foundation and freedom to make my dreams a reality. I cherish your love and belief in me. Thank you from the bottom of my heart.

About the Author

Linda J. Curry is an author, speaker and teacher in the areas of spiritual, emotional, and physical well-being. Dedicated to living her best life, Linda assists others with cultivating health through her expertise in spiritual growth, herbalism, plant-based culinary cuisine, and coaching.

Gifted in healthy food preparation, she spends much of her time simplifying nutrition for individuals and groups, teaching them how to cleanse and nourish the body through whole plant cuisine. In addition to being a health foodie and vegetable advocate, Linda utilizes a variety of wellness approaches to balance her life and enjoys sharing her wisdom with others.

Linda has worked as a raw food chef at an alternative cancer clinic in Mesa, Arizona and featured her skills as a plant-based chef on ABC's Sunday morning show in Phoenix, Arizona. In addition, she established a two-year Meatless Monday's luncheon from 2012 – 2014 encouraging others to improve their health as well as making a positive impact on global warming. She sells her recipe books at www.TrueBalanceWellness.com as well as a natural skin-care line where she offers her own handcrafted medicinal salves, facial creams, deodorant, oils and more.

Linda lives in Mesa, Arizona with her husband, Rich, and their beloved cat, Gracie Mae. They have deep respect for the earth and try to live as sustainably as they can. They have co-created a sacred space at home with many friends such as coyotes, javelina, rabbits, owls, bobcats, quail, rattlesnakes, scorpions and more. They grow much of their own food, attempting to keep the wildlife out of the garden. Linda enjoys spending time with her extended family as well including her nieces and nephews who continue to remind her how precious life is and to embrace each moment.